MEDITERRANEAN DIET

The Complete Mediterranean Diet Cookbook for Beginners. Quick Recipes and Easy Meal Plans for Healthy Weight Loss. Change Your Eating Habits and Live Well Every Day Fighting Diabetes

DIRTY MOORE

CONTENTS

Part III - Plan

INTRODUCTION

The food and culture are interwoven inseparably. We learn what good food is from the elders, who have in turn learned the same thing themselves from the previous generation. In this way, national recipes and tastes are both acquired and inherited, becoming an integral part of the cultural identity, something that we carry within us no matter where we end up living. Some families go so far as to have their own twists and tweaks of the traditional dishes that are jealously guarded against all foreigners. Through the wonders of modern mobility, cultures combine like never before and different dishes meld, creating something completely unique and endemic. The Western countries are a wonderful example of national cuisines from all over the world coming together in a single crock pot. Seeing a string of national restaurants right in the middle of a modern metropolis such as Munich is by now a completely ordinary sight, but the fact that one can order and simultaneously eat authentic kebabs and gyros is simply amazing. No matter how different they are, these various dishes still share a common ancestry, one which has been pinpointed as originating from the area roughly surrounding the Mediterranean Sea.

The Mediterranean diet is all about living well and eating like the people of the Mediterranean. This includes vegetables, grains, legumes, dairy, eggs, poultry and smaller amounts of red meat. It's about dining with friends, moderate physical activity, and food that will lift your spirits. It's all about eating the traditional food of the countries that make up the Mediterranean, including Italy,

Spain, France, Greece, Israel, and even Turkey. This diet promotes overall health, including weight loss, and it's great at helping reduce the risk of Parkinson's, Alzheimer's, promoting heart health, and reducing the risk of cancer.

If you want to lose weight, simply eat less than you expend, and voila! Don't eat junk food, eat everything in moderation, and you're good! Less frying, more veggies, no snacks. Easy-peasy! Or, is it? As someone who, much like yourself, struggled to lose weight for a long time, I have something to admit. I hated diet manuals and cookbooks. The majority I came across gave a lot of useful information, but none told me how to really apply them. I read countless seemingly healthy recipes only to discover that creating the meals took a lot of time, not including the hours spent every week just to make sure my fridge and pantry were well-stocked. In the meantime, I'd go hungry when none of the ingredients were in my fridge, and, with no time to go out and shop for groceries, I'd just eat the first thing that was fastest to cook.

With the Mediterranean Diet you'll have foods that are based on vegetable, fruits, grains, olive oil, nuts, beans, legumes, herbs, spices and seeds. You'll consume fish and seafood often, with cheese, yogurt and other dairy products in moderation. Poultry and eggs are allowed in moderation, but you shouldn't eat them more than twice a week. Other meats and sweets should be eaten rarely, and drinking water is encouraged. Say goodbye to sodas and replace it with a glass of red wine in the evenings and water to hydrate. While physical activity isn't required on this diet, at least moderate activity is encouraged if you to get the most out of the Mediterranean lifestyle. Even taking an evening stroll can help to elevate the effects of the diet, including weight loss.

THE MEDITERRANEAN DIET AS A FOOD MODEL

If you are searching for a healthy way to lose the weight and to maintain an optimal health, then this is the best diet for you. It's the Mediterranean diet, a very popular and unique one. When talking about the Mediterranean diet, it is necessary to emphasize that its pattern follows one of the healthiest diets worldwide. The best way to know something is to live it, so we recommend that you sign up for the Mediterranean diet and discover why it is the perfect diet for yourself.

The Mediterranean diet is mainly based on the foods people from countries like Italy and Greece used to eat back in the '60s. Researches in the field proved that these were extremely healthy and that they had a very low risk of many illnesses. Besides the fact that the Mediterranean diet can help you lose the extra weight, it can also prevent the appearance of heart related illnesses, strokes and even diabetes.

This healthy lifestyle is based on consuming easy to find products that are full of important nutrients, vitamins and antioxidants. All these contribute to a healthy body and appearance. The Mediterranean lifestyle encourages physical exercise and enjoying the meals you make with friends and family. The diet has few limitations and it allows a lot of experimentation with ingredients and flavors. Now that you are familiarized with this diet and with its main principles, it's time you knew what you can and cannot eat. Basically, you can eat all kinds of vegetables, nuts, seeds, fruits, whole, grains, legumes, herbs, fish, seafood and healthy foods. Always avoid sodas, candies, ice cream, white bread, refined wheat, margarines and other trans fats, canola oil, soybean oil, hot dogs and anything labeled low-fat or diet.

These are the main products you can and cannot consume during the Mediterranean diet, but we thought you could use more specific guidelines as well. Therefore, here are the ingredients you should base your Mediterranean diet meals on! When it comes to veggies, there are a lot of options. You can eat tomatoes, eggplants, kale, broccoli, spinach, cauliflower, cucumbers, avocados, carrots, Brussels sprouts, parsnips, turnips, artichokes, endives, fennels, etc.

As far as fruits are concerned, feel free to eat as many apples, oranges, pears, bananas, grapes, strawberries, blueberries, blackberries, melons, peaches, apricots, figs or dates as you like. Also, you can consume walnuts, almonds, hazelnuts, pumpkin seeds, sunflower seeds, cashews, macadamia nuts, chia seeds, hemp seeds, etc.

Make sure your meals also contain peas, all kind of beans, chickpeas, peanuts, lentils. Don't forget you can make delicious meals using yams, sweet potatoes and regular potatoes. Whole oats, rice, rye, barley, corn, whole wheat, quinoa and bulgur are also a must if following the Mediterranean diet.

As a basis of Mediterranean Diet, it's highly recommended a green leaf before each meal. Raw plant foods mean in their interpretation of "live" food, which in nature contains all the vital substances for the body. In addition, raw food is given even greater importance in the prevention of health and the treatment of disease. Due to the content of ballast substances, raw food stimulates regular stools, while refined and denatured food is often the cause of constipation—a widespread and far from harmless affliction today. An extremely important property of raw food is its beneficial effect on metabolic processes. Raw food increases the speed of their flow and stimulates a thorough cleaning of the body from toxins and poisons, thereby increasing its defenses. Introduction to the diet of raw plant food in sufficient volume is of great importance for the heart and blood vessels, since such food normalizes the level of Fat in the blood and largely counteracts the tendency to clotting blood that appears after traditional meals. This makes the daily intake of raw plant foods before each meal indispensable in the prevention of health. In general, raw food should be in the daily diet 30-50%.

BENEFITS OF THE MEDITERRANEAN DIET

The Mediterranean diet's impact on heart health is one of its most commonly studied aspects, and there is copious research demonstrating its positive effect on coronary and vascular function.

As you can see, the health benefits of the Mediterranean diet have been widely and comprehensively studied. Again, and again, the Mediterranean diet is found to be an excellent way to improve heart, bone, and overall health and reduce the risk of cardiovascular disease, type 2 diabetes, metabolic syndrome, and some types of cancer.

The fact that it's a delicious way to eat that can also help you lose weight just makes the Mediterranean diet that much more appealing!

A Delicious Path to Weight Loss

One of the best ways to ensure that a diet will help you reach your weight-loss goals is to choose one that allows you to eat a wide variety of delicious foods and doesn't require you to go hungry, do without all of your favorite treats, or buy a lot of expensive and obscure ingredients. This is where the Mediterranean diet really stands out. There are no strict rules to follow and there is no deprivation or any need to drive all over town hunting down exotic ingredients or expensive supplements.

Heart health

Research shows that greater compliance with the traditional Mediterranean diet, which includes monounsaturated and omega-3 Fatty acids, is associated with a significant reduction in mortality, especially heart disease.

Olive oil is also beneficial for reducing hypertension because nitric oxide is more bioavailable, allowing it to dilate blood vessels and keep it clean. Another element of protection is that it helps to combat the effects of oxidation that promotes disease and improves endothelial function. People in the Mediterranean generally have no difficulty maintaining healthy cholesterol levels because they eat lots of healthy

Keeps your heart healthy and reduces risk factors of cardiovascular heart disease. There are many factors of the Mediterranean diet that improve heart health such as the addition of olive oil and wine. Olive oil is high in alpha-linolenic acid (ALA) which has been found to decrease the risk of cardiac or premature death by almost 30%. Compared to other oils like sunflower oil or vegetable oil, only olive oil has been found to significantly lower blood pressure. With a healthier diet focused on good fats, the Mediterranean diet can also maintain the HDL cholesterol in the body, the "good" cholesterol, and decrease the LDL "bad" cholesterol. Not only that, but it also reduces the level of unhealthy fatty triglycerides in the blood. A high level of these has been linked to an increased risk of stroke or sudden cardiac death. With the improvement of these risk factors, the body can have better blood flow and fewer plaque build-ups which keeps the arteries open and blood steadily pumping throughout the body. A study found that when obese men followed the Mediterranean diet, they had better blood flow compared to when they ate junk food and their arteries did not dilate.

Protection From Diseases

Improves the longevity of your life. We have no guarantee of our future, but the research shows that the Mediterranean lifestyle may have the ability to increase your life span. A famous study called the Lyon Diet Heart Study followed patients who had suffered from heart attacks between 1988 and 1992. They were told to follow either a normal post-heart attack low-fat diet recommended by doctors at the time or the Mediterranean diet. Nearly 4 years after the study started, researchers found that the group who followed the Mediterranean diet had nearly 70% less risk of heart disease and 50% less risk of death than the followers of the low-fat diet. This longevity was also very much visible in the people of the Mediterranean that Ancel Keys first studied when he found the link between diet and quality of life. With all the benefits of the Mediterranean diet in improving your health, such as reducing the risk of cancer, heart disease, and neurodegenerative diseases, it's only logical that this will keep you healthy for longer. All by simply changing the types of food you're eating! Fresh fruits and vegetables tend to contain higher antioxidants which are great for strengthening your immune system and preventing disease.

Diabetes

Nutrition researchers have repeatedly found associations between lower rates of type 2 diabetes and this diet. In some of the most compelling trials, published in 2018 in Nutrition & Diabetes, researchers compared a low-fat diet to the much higher-fat Mediterranean Diet and found that, among other health indicators, diabetes rates were lower in people eating the Mediterranean Diet.

Reduces your risk of having Type 2 diabetes. For people who have a family history of diabetes or who struggle with unstable blood sugar levels, this type of diabetes can feel imminent in their future. But the Mediterranean diet has been able to lessen the chances of acquiring diabetes (Type 2) because of its healthy eating patterns and allowing you to lose extra weight. Studies have shown that patients can lose more weight following the Mediterranean diet than other low Carb or low-fat diet plans. This is a great way to reduce your risk of diabetes because extra weight is always a risk factor. Patients have seen improvements in their blood sugar levels and even been able to change their medication dosage or quit it entirely! This diet encourages the consumption of fibrous foods like whole grains, beans, legumes, and fresh vegetables. When the body has enough fiber, it's able to slow digestion and make you feel full for a longer period of time. This minimizes the need for frequent snacking which is what can cause blood sugar spikes every time you eat. This means less insulin is produced. The Mediterranean diet doesn't follow a low carbohydrate philosophy, but it cuts foods that cause blood sugar spikes from your diet such as sugary snacks, refined grains, and soda.

Prostate Cancer, 'Whole' Mediterranean Diet Could Reduce Your Risk

There is a lot of research yet to cover in the area of cancer prevention, but some tentative research has labeled the Mediterranean diet has one of the best environments to combat cancer cells. A 2013 Italian research study found that the Mediterranean diet provided the highest levels of fiber, antioxidants, and omega 3 fatty acids compared to other diets. With the high intake of fruits, olive oil, fish, whole grains, vegetables, and wine, you're eating healthier, natural foods and avoiding the garbage of processed foods, trans fats, and sugar. It's important to note that diet only goes so far and this information is in the very beginning phases. You should always go for cancer screenings and annual health exams.

Weight Loss In Obesity

Despite all the diet strategies out there, weight management still comes down to "calories in versus calories out." Fad diets may promise that avoiding carbs or eating a soup full of cabbage is the secret to losing weight, but if you want to shed those pounds, it ultimately comes down to eating fewer calories than you burn.

Cognitive Ability

Improves mental focus and cognitive functioning. Omega 3 fatty acids are composed of two parts: DHA and EPA. Along with vision health, as we mentioned above, they are also vital in brain development and functioning. They help preserve the health of brain cells and improve the communication between brain cells to allow for faster neural communication. As we get older, our brain is affected by natural signs of aging which can lead to the destruction of neural cells and neurodegenerative diseases like Alzheimer's, dementia, and Parkinson's. The omega 3 fatty acids of the Mediterranean diet are loaded with substances to protect the brain from premature aging and decline in functioning. Along with healthy fruits and vegetables, and removing processed foods and sugars from your diet, you can improve your memory recall, mental focus, and overall cognitive functioning.

Major Depressive Disorder

According to a study, those who follow the Mediterranean diet can help reduce the risk of depression. Researchers participating in the study examined the mental health effects of adherence to various diets, such as the Mediterranean diet, the Healthy Eating Index (HEI) diet, Dietary approaches to stop hypertension (DASH diet), and the rate of inflammation of the diet. They found that the risk of depression decreased further when people followed a traditional Mediterranean diet and generally ate various anti-inflammatory foods.

Could lower the risk of mental illnesses like depression and anxiety. Other areas where more research is necessary is in mental illnesses. Some research has linked depression, obsessive-compulsive disorder, and anxiety to high amounts of inflammation in the body. With the Mediterranean diet, you're eating high-quality foods that prevent inflammation. Fish and plant-based foods, in particular, have great anti-inflammatory properties, as well as the wine you're encouraged to drink in moderation.

Helps To Prevent Frailty

A diet rich in fresh plant-based foods and healthy Fats is a winning combination for long life. Monounsaturated

Fatty acids, found in olive oil and some nuts, are the main source of Fat in the Mediterranean diet. Time and time again, studies have shown that monounsaturated Fats are associated with low levels of heart disease, cancer, depression, cognitive diseases, Alzheimer's, inflammatory diseases, etc. Currently, heart disease is by far the leading cause of death in developed countries.

Anti-Inflammatory

Can clear acne breakouts and improve the look and health of your skin. Any dermatologist will tell you that sugar is bad for your skin and can cause pimples or acne breakouts. Not only that, it can destroy the natural collagen present under your skin which is what gives skin that youthful elasticity. The Mediterranean diet can help skin healthy two-fold: by having a diet rich in fruits and vegetables with natural antioxidants to keep the skin healthy, and by avoiding processed sugar that is found in baked goods and candy. The natural sugars found in fruit are not harmful to the body compared to refined sugar which can cause blood sugar spikes followed by skin irritations. Studies have found that when adult women who did not consume enough fish or fresh fruits and vegetables a week had nearly double the risk of having adult acne.

YOUR BODY CHANGES WITH THE MEDITERRANEAN DIET

The Mediterranean diet is inspired by the eating habits of the populations that around the Mediterranean Sea. The populations of southern Italy and Greece are the main regions that influence this diet. But, it isn't the diet that is consumed today in many of these regions that gained so much attention. The Mediterranean diet refers to the traditional eating habits and lifestyles of these areas in the 1950s and 1960s. It was during this time that researchers noticed a significant difference in the health of populations in these areas when compared to those living in America. It was obvious that many of the individuals in the Mediterranean areas were healthier and the key difference between those living in the Mediterranean and those living in America was their diet.

If you decide to follow the Mediterranean diet, the establishment of your diet will be natural products, vegetables, entire grain pieces of bread, pasta, rice, grains, and potatoes, alongside beans, nuts, vegetables, and seeds. These foods ought to be consumed day by day and will shape the premise of each meal you eat, with crisp vegetables becoming the overwhelming focus. While carbohydrates are a piece of this diet, they will, in general, be entire, unpredictable, high in fiber, and consumed with protein or fats simultaneously.

Fish and seafood are the staple proteins in this diet. Ordinary consumption of greasy fish, similar to salmon, mackerel, and fish, assists with satiety as well as lifts admission of heart solid omega-3 unsaturated fats. When looking for fish, be that as it may, avoid ranch-raised at whatever point conceivable. Extra wellsprings of fat incorporate olive and canola oil, which replace margarine and grease for cooking and dressing food. With some restraint, you'll eat poultry, eggs, cheddar, and plain, unsweetened yoghurt each other day or a couple of times each week relying upon your inclination. Decide on characteristic dairy and cheddar, not vigorously handled or seasoned assortments, to avoid added additives, sugars, or synthetics. Goat cheddar and feta cheddar are normally observed on Mediterranean diet menus. Desserts, for example, crude nectar, are appreciated in exacting control, while different treats are eaten distinctly on extraordinary events. Red meat is barely consumed in the Mediterranean diet, alongside exceptionally handled meats like wieners and bacon. On the in addition to side, a solitary glass of wine is considered a staple in the diet and part of what makes the diet so heart solid, so don't feel awful about presenting yourself with a glass with your supper.

Who This Diet Is Well Suited For?

This diet will work well for someone who wants to boost their heart well-being, reduce their cholesterol, lose some weight, and do without feeling insulted as such. Note, though, if you consume too many processed grains in your diet (white breads, white pasta, and so on), this will potentially build up your cholesterol level, so it's important to concentrate on healthier grains that have been handled as poorly as you would expect under the circumstances. This diet is likewise extraordinary for the individuals who don't react well to a conventional low carb diet. A significant piece of the Mediterranean diet is the worth set on regular exercise, which is bolstered by the vitality you'll get from complex carbohydrates and common natural product sugars. Try not to be amazed if 50-60% of your all-out everyday calorie consumption originates from carbohydrates while on this plan. At last, the plan is extraordinary for the individuals who are hoping to keep up their weight utilizing a dietary convention that can be supported for quite a long time to come. Since you are not dispensing with any food bunches altogether, it's truly conceivable to get balanced nutrition with this plan.

HOW DOES MEDITERRANEAN DIET WORK?
DIETARY COMPONENTS

This healthy lifestyle is based on consuming easy to find products that are full of important nutrients, vitamins and antioxidants. All these contribute to a healthy body and appearance.

Some of the great things about this excellent diet is that it's not costly. It's really a budget friendly one that uses affordable ingredients that anyone can afford.

The Mediterranean lifestyle encourages physical exercise and enjoying the meals you make with friends and family.

The diet has few limitations and it allows a lot of experimentation with ingredients and flavors.

Now that you are familiarized with this diet and with its main principles, it's time you knew what you can and cannot eat.

Basically, you can eat all kinds of vegetables, nuts, seeds, fruits, whole, grains, legumes, herbs, fish, seafood and healthy foods.

You should consume in moderation eggs, poultry, pork, cheese, sour cream, heavy cream and yogurt and you should almost never eat beef.

You should never eat processed meat, sweetened beverages, refined oil or processed foods.

Whole oats, rice, rye, barley, corn, whole wheat, quinoa and bulgur are also a must if following the Mediterranean diet.

Last but not least, consume shrimp, clams, crab, mussels, sardines, salmon, tuna, trout, mackerel or oysters.

Consume chicken, duck, turkey, pork, lamb, eggs, cheese, yogurt and Greek yogurt as well.

Season your foods with salt, pepper, garlic, mint, basil, sage, rosemary, nutmeg, cinnamon, saffron, turmeric, cumin, peppercorns, fennel seeds, etc.

Use healthy oils like avocado or olive oil ones.

If you decide that the Mediterranean lifestyle suits you, make sure you drink enough water during the day. You can also drink moderate amounts of wine (mostly red wine), coffee and tea. Just make sure that you don't consume sweetened beverages and fruits juices that contain a lot of sugar.

Snacks should be included in a Mediterranean diet plan. Some great snack ideas would be a serving of nuts, fruits like plums and grapes, dried fruits like apricots, hummus with veggie sticks or mashed avocado on whole wheat toast. Now that you know what you can eat on a Mediterranean diet, it's time to find out which foods you have to avoid.

First of all, red meat shouldn't be an option on a Mediterranean diet. You will have to avoid beef as much as possible. Also, try to limit the consumption of processed meat like sausages or salami.

Avoid added sugars if you want to stick to your healthy diet. This means you have to stay away from candy, baked goods and sweetened drinks like soda.

Use honey, stevia and even cinnamon to sweeten your desserts, tea and coffee.

Make sure you don't use white flour or refined grains like white rice. These have a lower nutritional value and they don't contain the fibers you need. You can replace them with brown rice, whole wheat grains and almond flour.

Last but not least, try to replace the butter with olive oil. This will suit the Mediterranean diet better.

As you can see, this diet doesn't have as many restrictions as you might think but these guidelines should be followed in order to enjoy the health benefits and weight loss.

The Mediterranean diet limits the meat consumption and is based on eating a lot of veggies and fruits. Therefore, this diet is suitable for vegans and vegetarians as well.

So, if you are a vegan who wants to start a Mediterranean diet you can consume nuts, seeds, tofu and even beans. It's actually pretty easy to follow this diet if you are a vegan. All you have to do is to focus on eating certain foods.

First of all, you can consume a lot of beans because they contain healthy proteins and fibers. They prevent the appearance of heart related issues and they are vital for such a diet. Use them to make salads, sautés, soups and stews.

You can also consume tofu as a meat replacement. Add small servings of tofu to your meals a few times per week.

Nuts and seeds are a great option if you are a vegan on a Mediterranean diet. They provide the omega-3 you need in order to stay healthy. include flaxseeds, walnuts, hemp seeds and chia seeds to your diet.

Also, add fibers and whole grains to you diet in order to feel full and satisfied longer. Eat more quinoa, whole wheat pasta and whole wheat bread.

Veggies are extremely important if you are a vegan following such a diet. Consume as many veggies as you like because they contain all the vitamins a vegan need.

If you are a vegan you can eat as many fruits as you like. These are not just healthy, but they can also satisfy your sweet tooth. Fruits like berries, oranges, grapefruits or raspberries contain a lot of vitamins and antioxidants and they should be included in your diet.

Last but not least, try to see this diet as a healthy lifestyle. Embrace it and make it your own. We guarantee it will soon show its amazing benefits.

The Mediterranean diet can change your life, it can definitely improve your healthy, your appearance and your metabolism. You simply must make sure you consume the foods allowed and that you avoid anything that can interfere with the success of this diet.

That's a simple formula of success and anyone can follow such a diet. It's not a complex one and it will make you feel so much different in no time.

If you made the decision to opt for the Mediterranean diet, you might need to know something more. There are some tips and tricks that will help you stay on your diet and enjoy it. Also, you might want to know what to include in your shopping list and what to eat when you go out with friends and you are on the Mediterranean diet.

While a great many people realize they ought to keep away from soft drinks and milkshakes, numerous individuals don't understand that even beverages publicized to support athletic execution or improve health can be stacked with undesirable fixings.

HOW TO BUILD A FOOD PLAN

Look for Short Ingredient List: The bulk of the food is listed in order according to weight and are usually the first ingredients. If you don't recognize an ingredient, place it back on the shelf! Consider using products that have no more than 5 ingredients. The longer ingredients probably are the result of unnecessary extras including artificial preservatives.

Check Serving Sizes: Packages often time contain more than a single serving. Visualize how many calories and the amount of sugar is in a single container. Thus, you need to check the serving size first.

Discover Calorie Counts: It is essential to check the labels calorie count since they are very important during your process using the Mediterranean diet plan.

Avoid Fats: It's important to remove foods from your diet plan that contain any fully hydrogenated or partially hydrogenated oils.

Check the Percent of Daily Value: The daily value will tell you how many nutrients are in each serving of a packaged item.

Get More Of These Nutrients: Look for calcium, iron, fiber, vitamin A, and vitamin C.

The Label Explained

· Serving Information At the Top: This provides the size of one serving and per container.

· Check the total calories per serving and container.

· Limit certain nutrients from your diet.

· Provide yourself with plenty of beneficial nutrients

· Understand the % of daily value section.

Avoid These Foods

· Added Sugar: Ice cream, candy, regular soda, plus many others.

· Trans fats: Found in various processed foods such as margarine, added sugar, ice cream, candies, table sugar, soda, and others. Added sugars, sugar-sweetened beverages, refined grains, processed meats, and other highly processed foods.

·   Processed Meat Products: Hot dogs, processed sausages, bacon
·   Refined Grains: Pasta made with refined wheat, white bread

Note If You Are Pregnant: You should avoid some of the oily fish such as swordfish, shark, and tuna because some may contain low levels of toxic heavy metals.

What to Eat Rarely:

·   Red meats (Limit to once each week)

Foods You Can Eat

Seafood and Fish: Mussels, clams, crab, prawns, oysters, shrimp, tuna, mackerel, salmon, trout, sardines, anchovies, and more

Poultry: Turkey, duck, chicken, and more

Eggs: Duck, quail, and chicken eggs

Dairy Products: Contain calcium, B12, and Vitamin A: Greek yogurt, regular yogurt, cheese, plus others

Tubers: Yams, turnips, potatoes, sweet potatoes, etc.

Vegetables: Another excellent choice for fiber, and antioxidants: Cucumbers, carrots, Brussels sprouts, tomatoes, onions, broccoli, cauliflower, spinach, kale, eggplant, artichokes, fennel, etc.

Seeds and Nuts: Provide minerals, vitamins, fiber, and protein: Macadamia nuts, cashews, pumpkin seeds, sunflower seeds, hazelnuts, chestnuts, Brazil nuts, walnuts, almonds, pumpkin seeds, sesame, poppy, and more

Fruits: Excellent choices for vitamin C, antioxidants, and fiber: Peaches, bananas, apples, figs, dates, pears, oranges, strawberries, melons, grapes, etc.

Spices and Herbs: Cinnamon, garlic, pepper, nutmeg, rosemary, sage, mint, basil, parsley, etc.

Whole Grains: Whole grain bread and pasta, buckwheat, whole

wheat, barley, corn, whole oats, rye, quinoa, bulgur, couscous

Legumes: Provide vitamins, fiber, carbohydrates, and protein: Chickpeas, pulses, beans, lentils, peanuts, peas

Healthy Fats: Avocado oil, avocados, and olives are excellent fats. The monounsaturated fat which is found in olive oil is a fat that can help reduce the 'bad' cholesterol. The oil has become the traditional fat worldwide with some of the healthiest populations. A great deal of research has been provided showing the oil is a huge plus towards the risk of heart disease because of the antioxidants and fatty acids.

You will still need to pay close attention when purchasing olive oil because it may have been extracted from the olives using chemicals or possibly diluted with other cheaper oils, such as canola and soybean. You need to be aware of refined or light olive or regular oils. The Mediterranean diet plan calls for the use of extra-virgin olive oil because it has been standardized for purity using natural methods providing the sensory qualities of its excellent taste and smell. The oil is high in phenolic antioxidants which makes—real—olive oil beneficial.

Beverage Options: Maintaining a healthy body requires plenty of water, and the Mediterranean diet plan is not any different. Tea and coffee are allowed, but you should avoid fruit juices or sugar-sweetened beverages that contain large amounts of sugar.

White Meats: White meats are high in minerals, protein, and vitamins but you should remove any visible fat and the skin.

Red Meats: You are allowed red meats including lamb, pork, and beef in small quantities. They are rich in minerals, vitamins, and protein—especially iron. Use caution because they do contain more fat—specifically saturated fat—compared to the fat content found in poultry. Don't leave it out entirely; save it for a special dinner or with a stew or casserole.

Potatoes: You have noticed that potatoes are listed in the tubers group because they are a healthy choice, but it will greatly depend on how they are prepared. You receive potassium, Vitamin B, Vitamin C, and some of your daily fiber nutrients. You must consider that they do contain large amounts of starch which can be quickly converted to glucose which can be harmful and place you at some risk of type 2 diabetes. Use simpler methods of cooking them including baking, boiling, and mashing them without butter.

Desserts and Sweets: Biscuits, cakes, and sweets should be consumed in small quantities, as a special treat. Not only is the sugar a temptation for type 2 diabetes; it can also promote tooth decay. Many times, they may also contain higher levels of saturated fats. You can receive some nutritional value, but as a general rule—stick to small portions.

What to Eat in Moderation: Eggs, poultry, milk, butter, yogurt, and cheese.

TIPS FOR GETTING STARTED

If you are choosing to drop the pounds and keep them off, you will discover the Mediterranean style is the cure you have been seeking. You have to get motivated to get any plan to work for you. The first step was taken since you purchased this informative guide.

Jot down your goals and the reasons you need to change your eating patterns. As you proceed with your weight loss, keep your motivation in check by referring to those reasons. It will give you a needed boost.

Surround yourself with people that are positive; you will develop emotionally healthy realistic goals. Dropping the pounds will be the result, but first, you need to set goals. You need to make the goals small with sustainable things that you have full control over to be successful. You can make simple goals such as how many servings of fruits you will eat in one day or how many hours of sleep you will have that night.

It is essential for you to recharge and take the evening hours to relax and improve your sleep hygiene. Try to leave work – at work. Deal with the issues when you return. If you are going through a tough time or working long hours, you tend to forget items you may 'munch' on as you are working. Make it a point to write down everything you eat.

Working long hours can be beneficial for knocking off those pounds, but it can also cause you to be restless and can lead to post-workout insomnia if you have worked out or done other strenuous physical activities on your evenings off.

No matter what the case, slow down for at least an hour or more before attempting to retire for the evening.

If you have dieted before, you already know you will reach spans of time where your weight loss will level out. That's merely a segment of weight loss that can't be moderated. All you need to do is remain consistent. The weight loss will return. It is much better to expect problems or roadblocks than it is to believe that the new dieting methods will be smooth sailing.

Set a timeline with realistic goals. Choosing to lose weight is a fantastic move, but you need to be realistic. You might find it helpful to use baby steps to achieve the desired goal. For example, set a goal to lose six pounds in the next five to six weeks when you begin your new Mediterranean diet plan. For most people, healthy benefits are received if you start the plan by losing five to ten percent of your starting weight. It may not be your ideal medically suggested weight, but it is going to lead you toward a healthier weight. Take baby steps.

Consider what you want to change about the way you feel concerning your weight issues. If you notice you are craving sweets, your plan should include a way to reduce your intake down to two times weekly. Provide you and your family with healthier, filling choices such as fruit. However, don't go cold turkey because the plan won't work. Search for a recipe that allows you to taste the sweetness without the additional calories.

After you have adjusted your body to the Mediterranean way of eating, be willing to change your goals as you make progress. By starting small, you leave the door open so you can make more significant challenges as you proceed through the plan.

If you're searching for the best tips on the most proficient method to get in shape and keep it off, this apparently interminable measure of counsel can be overpowering and confounding.

From the diets elevating crude foods to dinner designs that rotate around shakes and prepackaged foods, another prevailing fashion diet appears to spring up each day.

The issue is, albeit prohibitive diets and disposal feast plans will in all likelihood bring about transient weight loss, the vast majority can't keep up them and wind up quitting inside half a month. Numerous individuals accept they should receive a thorough exercise routine to kick off weight loss.

While different kinds of movement are significant when you're endeavoring to get fit as a fiddle, strolling is an astounding and simple approach to consume calories.

Actually, only 30 minutes of strolling every day has been appeared to help in weight loss.

Furthermore, it's an agreeable action that you can do both inside and outside whenever of day.

The genuine key to sheltered and effective weight loss is to embrace a healthy lifestyle that suits your individual needs and that you can keep up forever.

The accompanying tips are healthy, practical approaches to get you in the groove again and headed towards your weight and wellness objectives.

HOW MUCH DOES MEDITERRANEAN DIET COST?

Not only is the Mediterranean diet safe and tasty, it can also be a very low-cost way to lose weight. Focus on consuming whole food (rather than processed) during the season and shopping in farmers' markets ensures that you'll be buying items at their peak of flavour and at the lowest prices. Because we all remember, an apple is cheaper than a raspberry in November, and tastes great, too!

When you buy safe and sufficient ingredients, you'll most certainly consume the right foods, and you'll probably stick on your diet. Now that you do know what to buy if you're on a Mediterranean diet, it's time to discover some easy tricks and tips that will make things easier. You will see the Mediterranean diet as a modern, balanced lifestyle that will change your look and enhance your health. You should enjoy your meals, play with ingredients, flavours and textures. This way you will get real Mediterranean culinary feasts.

If you cannot find such products for sale or they are very expensive, then I suggest purchasing a special small mill for the coarse grinding of grain. Such a "semi-natural farm" will definitely be more economically advantageous than the purchase of similar products in super and hypermarkets or in specialized health food stores. True, in the consumption of grain should—as in everything else—abide by the measure. They acidify the body, their frequent consumption of canned food, under certain circumstances, increase susceptibility to disease.

The Mediterranean eating routine is the name that has been given to a specific dietary routine that was initially utilized by individuals in less fortunate areas of Italy and Greece for a long time. This eating routine was not initially thought to be especially sound in these areas, as the individuals ate these nourishments due to need, instead of in light of the Mediterranean eating routine weight reduction and fantastic sustenance benefits they encountered. This sort of food is far not quite the same as what you may anticipate from this district. However, it is generally a lot more advantageous in light of the fact that things like grease and margarine are seldom utilized.

The Mediterranean diet is a method for eating and a lifestyle shared by the individuals of the Mediterranean locale. Every one of the 16 countries that make up the Mediterranean coast feed also, in spite of the fact that they may offer some various highlights relying upon the area and culture.

As a general concept, the Mediterranean diet is characterized by the abundance and decent plant variety (e.g., natural products, fruits, peas, and tomatoes), olive oil consumption for preparing and seasoning, seafood, low-fat dairy, and moderate wine use. Due to the solid standing that the people of this place seemed to enjoy, with a presumed lower prevalence of some diseases, benefits offered by the Mediterranean diet have been foreseen in the course of the only remaining century. The properties of this diet have been identified by a foreign researcher in this district who has learned how to see the benefits of this style of eating.

MEDITERRANEAN BREAKFAST, LUNCH, DINNER AND SNACK RECIPES

Quick and easy recipes for weight loss

Baked Chicken in Under 30 Minutes

Preparation Time: 10 minutes

Cooking Time: 15 minutes

Servings: 3

Ingredients:

1 tbsp of EVOO

1 pound of boneless chicken breast (2 medium chicken breasts)

½ tsp of sea salt

¼ tsp of freshly ground pepper

¼ tsp of onion powder

¼ tsp of garlic powder

¼ tsp of paprika or red cayenne pepper

Directions:

Turn on the oven to 450 degrees Fahrenheit. Prepare the chicken for the dish and pour olive oil in a 10-inch baking dish. Pour oil on the chicken and coat it well and then place each piece of chicken side by side. In a mixing together, toss garlic powder, paprika, salt and pepper, and onion powder together. Season the chicken with the mixture on both sides until it coats it nicely and then bake for 15-20 minutes until the meat has reached a temperature of 165-170 degrees. It could take longer, if the chicken is bigger. Allow it to stand for 5-8 minutes before serving.

Serve hot with rice, noodles, or bread.

Nutrition: Calories: 215 Fat: 9g Carbs:1 g Protein:10 g

Spinach And Lentils Stew

Preparation Time: 10 minutes

Cooking Time: 20 minutes

Servings: 3

Ingredients:
   1 teaspoon olive oil
   1/3 cup brown lentils
   1 teaspoon ginger, grated
   4 garlic cloves, minced
   1 green chili pepper, chopped
   2 tomatoes, chopped
   ½ teaspoon turmeric powder
   2 potatoes, cubed
   A pinch of black pepper
   ¼ teaspoon cinnamon powder
   1 cup low-sodium veggie stock
   6 ounces spinach leaves

Directions:

Heat up a pot with the oil over medium heat, add chili pepper, ginger and garlic, stir and cook for 3 minutes.

Add tomatoes, pepper, cinnamon, turmeric, lentils, potatoes, stock and spinach, stir and cook for 20 minutes.

Divide into bowls and serve.

Nutrition:
   Calories: 220
   Protein: 11 g
   Fat: 3 g
   Carbs: 16 g

Cinnamon Apple and Lentils Porridge

Preparation Time: 5 minutes

Cooking Time: 10 minutes

Servings: 4

Ingredients:

½ cup walnuts, chopped

2 green apples, cored, peeled and cubed

3 tablespoons maple syrup

3 cups almond milk

½ cup red lentils

½ teaspoon cinnamon powder

½ cup cranberries, dried

1 teaspoon vanilla extract

Directions:

Put the milk in a pot, heat it up over medium heat, add the walnuts, apples, maple syrup and the rest of the ingredients, toss, simmer for 10 minutes, divide into bowls and serve.

Nutrition:

Calories 150

Fat 2 g

Fiber 1 g

Carbs 3 g

Protein 5 g

Grapes, Cucumbers and Almonds Soup

Preparation time: 10 minutes

Cooking time: 0 minutes

Servings: 4

Ingredients:

¼ cup almonds, chopped and toasted

3 cucumbers, peeled and chopped

3 garlic cloves, minced

½ cup warm water

6 scallions, sliced

¼ cup white wine vinegar

3 tablespoons olive oil

Salt and white pepper to the taste

1 teaspoon lemon juice

½ cup green grapes, halved

Directions:

In your blender, combine the almonds with the cucumbers and the rest of the ingredients except the grapes and lemon juice, pulse well and divide into bowls.

Top each serving with the lemon juice and grapes and serve cold.

Nutrition:

Calories 200

Fat 5.4

Fiber 2.4

Carbs 7.6

Protein 3.3

Tomato Bruschetta

Preparation time: 10 minutes

Cooking time: 10 minutes

Servings: 6

Ingredients:

1 baguette, sliced

1/3 cup basil, chopped

6 tomatoes, cubed

2 garlic cloves, minced

A pinch of salt and black pepper

1 teaspoon olive oil

1 tablespoon balsamic vinegar

½ teaspoon garlic powder

Cooking spray

Directions:

Arrange the baguette slices on a baking sheet lined with parchment paper, grease them with cooking spray and bake at 400° F for 10 minutes.

In a bowl, mix the tomatoes with the basil and the remaining ingredients, toss well and leave aside for 10 minutes.

Divide the tomato mix on each baguette slice, arrange them all on a platter and serve.

Nutrition:

Calories 265

Fat 18 g

Fiber 1 g

Carbs 21 g

Protein 10 g

Skillet Cod with Fresh Tomato Salsa

Preparation time: 20 minutes

Cooking time: 8 minutes

Servings: 4

Ingredients:

3 tomatoes, finely chopped

1 green bell pepper, finely chopped

¼ red onion, finely chopped

¼ cup pitted, chopped green olives

2 tablespoons white wine vinegar

1 tablespoon chopped fresh basil

½ teaspoon minced garlic

4 (4-ounce) cod fillets

Sea salt

Freshly ground black pepper

1 tablespoon olive oil

Directions:

In a small bowl, stir together the tomatoes, bell pepper, onion, olives, vinegar, basil, and garlic until well mixed. Set aside.

Season the fish with salt and pepper.

In a large skillet, heat the olive oil over medium-high heat. Pan-fry the fish, turning once, until it is just cooked through, about 4 minutes per side.

Transfer to serving plates and top with a generous scoop of tomato salsa.

Nutrition:

Calories: 181; Total fat: 7g; Saturated fat: 1g; Carbohydrates: 9g; Sugar: 4g; Fiber: 3g; Protein: 22g

EASY RECIPES FOR AWAY FROM HOME

Greek Style Spring Soup

Preparation Time: 10 minutes

Cooking time: 20 minutes

Servings: 4

Ingredients:
  3 cups chicken stock
  ½ pound chicken breast, shredded
  1 tablespoon chives, chopped
  1 egg, whisked
  ½ white onion, diced
  1 bell pepper, chopped
  1 tablespoon olive oil
  ¼ cup arborio rice
  ½ teaspoon salt
  1 tablespoon fresh cilantro, chopped

Directions:
  Pour olive oil in the stock pan and preheat it.

  Add onion and bell pepper. Roast the vegetables for 3-4 minutes. Stir them from time to time.

  After this, add rice and stir well.

  Cook the ingredients for 3 minutes over the medium heat.

  Then add chicken stock and stir the soup well.

  Add salt and bring the soup to boil.

  Add shredded chicken breast, cilantro, and chives. Add egg and stir it carefully.

  Close the lid and simmer the soup for 5 minutes over the medium heat. Remove the cooked soup from the heat.

Nutrition: Calories 176

Fat 5.6 g Fiber 7.6g Carbs 23.6 g Protein 4.6 g

Shredded Chicken Soup

Preparation Time: 10 minutes

Cooking time: 15 minutes

Servings: 4

Ingredients:

  3 cups chicken stock

  1-pound chicken breast, shredded

  ½ teaspoon dried mint

  ½ cup Greek yogurt

  ½ onion, diced

  1 tablespoon butter

  ½ teaspoon salt

  ½ teaspoon ground black pepper

  1 tablespoon fresh dill, chopped

Directions:

  Pour chicken stock in the saucepan and bring it to boil.

  Add shredded chicken, dried mint, salt, and ground black pepper.

  Simmer the liquid for 5 minutes over the low heat.

  Meanwhile, toss the butter in the skillet and melt it.

  Add onion and roast it until it is light brown.

  Add the cooked onion in the soup.

  Then add yogurt and stir it well.

  Bring the soup to boil, add dill, and remove from the heat.

  The soup is cooked.

Nutrition:

  Calories 198

  Fat 5.6 g   Fiber 7.6g   Carbs 23.6 g   Protein 4.6 g

Tomatillo Soup

Preparation Time: 10 minutes

Cooking time: 30 minutes

Servings: 4

Ingredients:

½ cup fresh coriander, chopped

2 cups tomatillos, chopped

1 white onion, diced

½ red onion, diced

2 bell peppers, chopped

1 tablespoon canola oil

1 tablespoon butter

½ teaspoon salt

½ teaspoon ground black pepper

3 cups of water

½ cup corn kernels

¼ cup green peas, frozen

Directions:

Pour canola oil in the skillet and preheat it.

Add chopped bell peppers and roast them for 5 minutes. Stir the vegetables from time to time. Meanwhile, toss the butter in the saucepan and melt it. Add tomatillos, white onion, and red onion.

Then add salt and ground black pepper and stir the vegetables.

Cook the vegetable mixture for 10 minutes over the medium heat. Stir them from time to time. After this, add cooked bell peppers in the saucepan. Add corn kernels and green peas. Then add water and coriander leaves. Stir the soup and bring it to boil. Simmer it for 10 minutes. With the help of the hand blender, blend the soup until you get a creamy texture.

Simmer the soup for 3 minutes over the high heat.

When the soup is cooked, let it rest for 10 minutes before serving.

Nutrition:

Calories 138

Fat 7.5

Fiber 4.1

Carbs 17.4

Protein 2.9

Kuru Fasulye

Preparation Time: 7 minutes

Cooking time: 55 minutes

Servings: 5

Ingredients:
  10 oz beef tenderloin

  1 ½ cup white beans

  6 cups of water

  1 teaspoon salt

  1 jalapeno pepper, chopped

  1 yellow onion, diced

  2 tablespoons avocado oil

  ½ teaspoon chili flakes

  1 tablespoon tomato paste

Directions:

Cut the beef tenderloin into the strips. After this, transfer the meat in the big saucepan. Add avocado oil and roast the meat for 5 minutes over the medium-high heat. Stir it from time to time.

Then add onion and jalapeno pepper. Stir it well and cook for 5 minutes more. After this, add white beans, tomato paste. Chili flakes, and salt. Add water and mix up the mixture until it will be homogenous and will get red color. Close the lid and cook the meal for 45 minutes over the medium-high heat. When the meal is cooked, all the ingredients will be tender.

Nutrition:
  Calories 338

  Fat 6.5

  Fiber 10.1 carbs 39.7

  Protein 31.1

Turmeric White Beans Soup

Preparation Time: 10 minutes

Cooking time: 50 minutes

Servings: 6

Ingredients:

   4 oz celery root, chopped

   1 cup white navy beans, dried

   5 cups chicken stock

   1 teaspoon turmeric

   1 yellow onion, diced

   1 tablespoon butter

   ½ cup fresh cilantro

   1 carrot, grated

   ¼ teaspoon minced garlic

   1 teaspoon tomato paste

   1 bay leaf

   1 teaspoon salt

   ½ teaspoon ground black pepper

   1 tablespoon fresh dill, chopped

Directions:

Pour chicken stock in the stock pan and add navy beans. Close the lid and cook them for 30 minutes over the high heat. Meanwhile, put the butter in the skillet and melt it. Add grated carrot and onion. Cook the vegetables until the onion is light brown. Then add celery root and roast the ingredients for 3 minutes more. Transfer the roasted vegetables in the stock pan. Then add bay leaf, tomato paste, minced garlic, salt, ground black pepper, and fresh dill. Add turmeric and stir the soup very carefully. Simmer it with the closed lid for 15 minutes more. The soup is cooked when the beans are tender.

Nutrition:

Calories 342 Fat 6.5 Fiber 10.1 Carbs 39.7 Protein 31.1

Instant Pot Beef Gyros

Preparation time: 10 minutes

Cook Time: 15 minutes

Servings: 6

Ingredients:

2 pounds beef roast, thinly sliced

1 tablespoon dried parsley

1 teaspoon salt

3 cloves minced garlic

1 teaspoon black pepper

1 sliced red onion

4 tablespoons oil of choice

1 teaspoon olive oil

½ cup vegetable broth

1 tablespoon lemon juice

For the Tzatziki sauce:

1 cup plain yogurt

1 clove minced garlic

2 tablespoon fresh dill

½ cup cucumber, peeled, seeded, and chopped finely

Directions:

Turn on instant pot and then add oil to the bottom.

Add meat, seasonings, garlic, and onion to sear and soften the onions. Pour the lemon juice and broth over meat, and then stir it, lock lid into place, and then use meat/stew and cook it for 9 minutes.

Let it natural release pressure for 3 minutes before quickly released.

Mix the Tzatziki sauce and if you want vegetable toppings or apple cider vinegar over this, you can. You can also put lettuce at the bottom of naan or pita bread before adding meat and toppings.

Nutrition: Calories: 395

Fat: 27g Carbs: 4gNet Carbs: 4g Protein: 32g Sodium 38%

Instant Pot Lasagna Hamburger Helper

Preparation time: 2 minutes

Cook Time: 5 minutes

Serves: 4

Ingredients:
- 1 box 16 oz, pasta
- 8 oz. Ricotta cheese
- ½ pound ground beef
- 1 jar pasta sauce
- 8 oz. Mozzarella cheese
- ½ pound ground sausage
- 4 cups water

Directions:

Put pot in sauté mood and cook meat till brown and crumbled.

Add in rest of ingredients, turn it on high pressure for five minutes.

Quick release it, and then put in half the cheese and half the mozzarella, and then put into a baking pan with more mozzarella. You can cook it for another 2-3 minutes till cheese melts.

Nutrition:
- Calories: 537
- Fat: 33g
- Carbs: 25 g
- Protein: 34g
- Fiber: 4g
- Sodium 36%

Grilled Fish with Lemons

Preparation Time: 5 Minutes

Cooking Time: 20 Minutes

Servings: 4

Ingredients:
   3-4 Lemons
   1 Tablespoon Olive Oil
   Sea Salt & Black Pepper to Taste
   4 Catfish Fillets, 4 Ounces Each
   Nonstick Cooking Spray

Directions:

Pat your fillets dry using a paper towel and let them come to room temperature. This may take ten minutes. Coat the cooking grate of your grill with nonstick cooking spray while it's cold. Once it's coated preheat it to 400 degrees.

Cut one lemon in half, setting it to the side. Slice your remaining half of the lemon into ¼ inch slices. Get out a bowl and squeeze a tablespoon of juice from your reserved half. Add your oil to the bowl, mixing well.

Brush your fish down with the oil and lemon mixture.

Place your lemon slices on the grill and then put our fillets on top. Grill with your lid closed. Turn the fish halfway through if they're more than a half an inch thick.

Nutrition:
   Calories: 147
   Protein: 22 Grams
   Fat: 1 Grams
   Carbs: 4 Grams
   Sodium: 158 mg

Pesto Walnut Noodles

Preparation Time: 5 minutes

Cooking Time: 25 minutes

Servings: 4

Ingredients:

    4 Zucchini, Made into Zoodles

    ¼ Cup Olive Oil, Divided

    ½ Teaspoon Crushed Red Pepper

    2 Cloves Garlic, Minced & Divided

    ¼ Teaspoon Black Pepper

    ¼ Teaspoon sea Salt

    2 Tablespoons Parmesan Cheese, Grated & Divided

    1 Cup Basil, Fresh & Packed

    ¾ Cup Walnut Pieces, Divided

Directions:

Start by making your zucchini noodles by using a spiralizer to get ribbons. Combine your zoodles with a minced garlic clove and tablespoon of oil. Season with salt and pepper and crushed red pepper. Set it to the side. Get out a large skillet and heat a ½ a tablespoon of oil over medium-high heat. Add in half of your zoodles, cooking for five minutes. You will need to stir every minute or so. Repeat with another ½ a tablespoon of oil and your remaining zoodles.

Make your pesto while your zoodles cook. Put your garlic clove, a tablespoon or parmesan, basil leaves and ¼ cup of walnuts in your food processor. Season with salt and pepper if desired and drizzle the remaining two tablespoons of oil in until completely blended.

Add the pesto to your zoodles, topping with remaining walnuts and parmesan to serve.

Nutrition:

    Calories: 301

    Protein: 7 Grams Fat: 28 Grams Carbs: 11 Grams Sodium: 160 mg

Tomato Tabbouleh

Preparation Time: 5 Minutes

Cooking Time: 30 Minutes

Servings: 4

Ingredients:

8 Beefsteak Tomatoes

½ Cup Water

3 Tablespoons Olive Oil, Divided

½ Cup Whole Wheat Couscous, Uncooked

1 ½ Cups Parsley, Fresh & Minced

2 Scallions Chopped

1/3 Cup Mint, Fresh & Minced

Sea Salt & Black Pepper to Taste

1 Lemon

4 Teaspoons Honey, Raw

1/3 Cup Almonds, Chopped

Directions:

Start by heating your oven to 400 degrees. Take your tomato and slice the top off each one before scooping the flesh out. Put the tops flesh and seeds in a mixing bowl.

Get out a baking dish before adding in a tablespoon of oil to grease it. Place your tomatoes in the dish, and then cover your dish with foil.

Now you will make your couscous while your tomatoes cook. Bring the water to a boil using a saucepan and then add the couscous in and cover. Remove it from heat and allow it to sit for five minutes. Fluff it with a fork.

Chop your tomato flesh and tops up, and then drain the excess water using a colander. Measure a cup of your chopped tomatoes and place them back in the mixing bowl. Mix with mint scallions, pepper, salt and parsley.

Zest your lemon into the bowl, and then half the lemon. Squeeze the lemon juice in and mix well.

Add your tomato mix to the couscous.

Carefully remove your tomatoes from the oven and then divide your tabbouleh among your tomatoes. Cover the pan with foil and then put it in the oven. Cook for another eight to ten minutes. Your tomatoes should be firm but still tender.

Drizzle with honey and top with almonds before serving.

Nutrition:
Calories: 314

Protein: 8 Grams

Fat: 15 Grams

Carbs: 41 Grams

Sodium: 141

PLAN FOR 28 DAYS

The 28-Day Plan

This will provide simple menus for the four weeks, as well as tips and guidelines on how to prep the food for each week. Rest assured, you don't need to be a gourmet chef to follow this plan, but you may want to make dishes ahead of time or chop your vegetables ahead of time—and I'll offer tips for streamlining the process. This part takes all the guesswork out of meal preparations.

I also give you easy and delicious snack ideas and suggested timing, as well as recommendations for how much water to drink. Your own "personal trainer" will offer a different workout for each week. You'll be able to track your patterns through an interactive chart that asks you to log your habits weekly.

The Mediterranean diet has quickly become one of the world's most popular and most effective diets, but it is more than an eating plan: The Mediterranean diet is a lifestyle. I will provide you with an overview of the Mediterranean diet and give you the information and tips you need to kick off your healthy journey and stay on it. From experimenting with new spices and ingredients to making time to enjoy a meal with your family, you will soon feel confident in your new Mediterranean lifestyle.

The Mediterranean diet plan is backed by science, and it's based in common sense—a variety of good whole foods with an emphasis on nutrition-dense foods. But to be successful, even the best diet requires commitment. Commitment is a huge factor when it comes to losing weight and keeping it off. This is a 28-day plan. Before you start it, take some time to fully commit to the time frame and the plan. Consider all the factors said so far, especially your habits and goals.

Every piece of this plan is equally important. The diet, the exercise, the charts, and the tips all go together to create the foundation of your journey to weight loss, weight maintenance, and overall good health.

The meal plans that follow are based on a 1,500- to 1,800-calorie-per-day diet. As you begin, it's important to follow the portions noted in the recipes (so if a recipe says it serves four, split it into four equal servings and only eat one). Everyone's individual caloric needs vary based on a number of metabolic factors and activity levels, so some people may discover the meal plans contain too many calories to lose weight. If this is the case for you, the following steps can help you adjust your calorie intake to a level that helps you lose weight:

Decrease portion size by one-fourth, so portions would be 75 percent of that listed in the recipes.

Increase activity levels.

Eat fewer and/or smaller snacks.

Conversely, if you exercise quite a bit and are losing more than a safe 1 to 2 pounds per week, add 3 ounces lean grilled protein to any vegetarian meals.

A NOTE ABOUT SNACKS: Snacks are okay—just make them count! This plan actually allows for two to three snacks per day if you are hungry. Suggested snacks are provided, but generally, snacks should include 1 ounce of protein—such as an ounce of nuts, two tablespoons of hummus, a tablespoon of nut butter; a half piece of fruit (or half cup of fruit such as berries); and either a cup of no starchy vegetables or a half cup of starchy vegetables.

WEEK 1
BREAKFAST

You might be following this plan to lose weight, or perhaps you just want to become healthier. Whatever your reason, this first week is all about first steps—and you may feel a mix of excitement and apprehension. This is natural. Once you go food shopping and tackle the prep work on a few recipes, you will feel better equipped to get through this toughest week. Take it one day at a time and be patient as you get into the swing of things. Remember your goals—post them or supportive words on your refrigerator as a reminder. If you are trying to lose weight, weigh yourself on the first day as a benchmark, but wait a week to weigh yourself again.

WEEK 1	BREAKFAST	LUNCH	DINNER
MONDAY	Savory Hummus Breakfast Toasts	Sirloin with Sweet Bell Peppers	North African Chicken Apricot Tagine
TUESDAY	Asparagus, Apple, and Feta Cheese Omelet	Quinoa and Spinach Salad with Figs and Balsamic Dressing	Oven-Roasted Puttanesca with Ground Beef
WEDNESDAY	Fresh Fruit Crumble Muesli	Greek-Style Tuna Salad in Pita	Balsamic-Basted Beef Kebabs with Barley and Spinach Risotto
THURSDAY	Greek Quinoa Breakfast Bowl	Delicious Broccoli Tortellini Salad	Spinach and Beans Mediterranean Style Salad
FRIDAY	Bulgur Fruit Breakfast Bowl	Chicken Drums With Peach Glaze	Lasagna
SATURDAY	Breakfast Egg on Avocado	Tuna and Cheese Bake	Teriyaki Chicken
SUNDAY	Breakfast Egg-artichoke Casserole	Instant Pot Potato Salad	Buffalo Chicken Quinoa Bowls

Savory Hummus Breakfast Toasts

Preparation Time: 10 minutes

Cooking Time: 3 minutes

Servings: 4

Ingredients:

4 multigrain bread slices

½ cup Traditional Hummus or store-bought hummus

½ cup sliced English cucumber

½ cup shredded carrot

¼ cup chopped oil-packed sun-dried tomatoes

1 scallion, both white and green parts, thinly sliced on the bias

¼ cup crumbled feta cheese

2 tablespoons sliced Kalamata olives

Directions:

Toast the bread and spread 2 tablespoons of hummus on each slice.

Divide the cucumber, carrot, sun-dried tomatoes, scallion, feta cheese, and olives between the toasts. Serve.

Nutrition:

Calories: 166

Total fat: 7g

Saturated fat: 2g

Carbohydrates: 20g

Sugar: 4g

Fiber: 5g

Protein: 8g

Asparagus, Apple, and Feta Cheese Omelet

Preparation Time: 20 minutes

Cooking Time: 20 minutes

Servings: 4

Ingredients:

2 tablespoons olive oil, divided

8 asparagus spears, chopped

1 garlic clove, minced

1 cup chopped spinach

¼ cup peeled chopped apple

1 tablespoon chopped fresh oregano

1 tablespoon chopped fresh basil

Sea salt

¼ cup chopped roasted red peppers

6 large eggs

¼ cup low-fat milk

⅓ cup crumbled feta cheese

Directions:

In a large skillet, heat 1 tablespoon of olive oil over medium heat. Cook the asparagus, stirring, for 4 to 5 minutes, until softened. Add the garlic and cook for 1 minute.

Add the spinach, apple, oregano, and basil. Season lightly with salt and continue cooking until the apples are softened and spinach has cooked down, about 5 minutes. Stir in the roasted red peppers and transfer the vegetables to a plate.

In a small bowl, whisk the eggs with the milk.

Wipe out the skillet, then heat the remaining 1 tablespoon of olive oil over medium heat and pour the eggs into the pan. As the eggs firm up, lift the edges and let the uncooked egg flow underneath, cooking until the eggs are almost set but still moist, 7 to 8 minutes. Season with salt.

Spoon the vegetable mixture onto one side of the omelet and sprinkle with the feta cheese. Fold the other half of the omelet over the cheese mixture and cook for 1 to 2 minutes more. Cut into slices and serve.

Nutrition:
Calories: 369
Total fat: 31g
Saturated fat: 12g
Carbohydrates: 7g
Sugar: 5g
Fiber: 2g
Protein: 17g

Fresh Fruit Crumble Muesli

Preparation Time: 20 minutes

Cooking Time: 0 minutes

Servings: 4

Ingredients:
   1 cup gluten-free rolled oats
   ¼ cup chopped pecans
   ¼ cup almonds
   4 pitted Medjool dates
   1 teaspoon vanilla extract
   ¼ teaspoon ground cinnamon
   1 cup sliced fresh strawberries
   1 nectarine, pitted and chopped
   2 kiwis, peeled and chopped
   ½ cup blueberries
   1 cup low-fat plain Greek yogurt

Directions:

In a food processor, combine the oats, pecans, almonds, dates, vanilla, and cinnamon and pulse until the mixture resembles coarse crumbs.

In a medium bowl, stir together the strawberries, nectarine, kiwis, and blueberries until well mixed. Divide the fruit and yogurt between bowls and top each bowl with the oat mixture. Serve.

Nutrition:
   Calories:258

Total fat: 6g
   Saturated fat: 0g
   Carbohydrates: 45g
   Sugar: 28g
   Fiber: 7g
   Protein: 11g

Greek Quinoa Breakfast Bowl

Preparation Time: 10 minutes

Cooking Time: 30 minutes

Servings: 6

Ingredients:

12 eggs

1 teaspoon onion powder

½ teaspoon salt

1 teaspoon olive oil

1-pint halved cherry tomatoes

2 cups cooked quinoa

¼ cup Greek yogurt, plain

1 teaspoon garlic powder

½ teaspoon black pepper

5 ounces of baby spinach

1 cup feta cheese

Directions:

Add the eggs into a bowl and whisk thoroughly. Combine the onion powder, garlic powder, Greek yogurt, pepper, and salt. Mix well.

Turn a stove burner to medium heat and place a large skillet on the burner. Allow it to heat up for about a minute. Pour in the olive oil and toss in the spinach. Cook for 3 to 4 minutes or until the spinach becomes wilted. Combine the cherry tomatoes into the skillet. Cook for another 3 minutes while stirring occasionally.

Add the eggs into the skillet and cook until they are set, which should take between 6 to 8 minutes. Stir the eggs often as you want them to look scrambled. Add in the feta and quinoa. Continue to cook the mixture until all the ingredients are cooked thoroughly. You can store this breakfast for four days in the fridge.

Nutrition:

Calories: 252 Fats: 16 g - Carbohydrates: 18 g - Protein: 10 g

Bulgur Fruit Breakfast Bowl

Preparation Time: 5 minutes

Cooking Time: 15 minutes

Servings: 6

Ingredients:

  2 cups 2% milk

  ½ teaspoon ground cinnamon

  1 ½ cups bulgur

  ½ cup almonds, chopped

  ½ cup mint, chopped (fresh is preferred)

  8 dried and chopped figs

  1 cup water

  2 cups frozen sweet cherries - you can also substitute in blueberries or blackberries

Directions:

Turn your stovetop to medium heat and combine the bulger, water, milk, and cinnamon. Lightly stir as the ingredients come to a boil.

Cover your mixture and turn the stove range temperature down to medium-low heat. Let the mixture simmer for 8 to 11 minutes. It is done simmering when about half of the liquid has been absorbed

Without removing the pan, turn off the range top heat and add the frozen cherries, almonds, and figs. Lightly stir and then cover for one minute so the cherries can thaw, and the mixture can combine.

Remove the cover and add in the mint before scooping your breakfast into a bowl.

Nutrition:

  Calories: 301,

  Fats: 6 Grams

  Carbohydrates: 57 Grams

  Protein: 9 Grams

Breakfast Egg on Avocado

Preparation Time: 3 minutes

Cooking Time: 15 minutes

Servings: 6

Ingredients:

1 tsp garlic powder

1/2 tsp sea salt

1/4 cup Parmesan cheese (grated or shredded)

1/4 tsp black pepper

3 medium avocados (cut in half, pitted, skin on)

6 medium eggs

Directions:

Prepare muffin tins and preheat the oven to 350oF.

To ensure that the egg would fit inside the cavity of the avocado, lightly scrape off 1/3 of the meat.

Place avocado on muffin tin to ensure that it faces with the top up.

Evenly season each avocado with pepper, salt, and garlic powder.

Add one egg on each avocado cavity and garnish tops with cheese.

Pop in the oven and bake until the egg white is set, about 15 minutes. Serve and enjoy.

Nutrition:

Calories per serving: 252

Protein: 14.0g

Carbs: 4.0g

Fat: 20.0g

Breakfast Egg-artichoke Casserole

Preparation Time: 35 minutes

Cooking Time: 35 minutes

Servings: 8

Ingredients:

16 large eggs

14 ounce can artichoke hearts, drained

10-ounce box frozen chopped spinach, thawed and drained well

1 cup shredded white cheddar

1 garlic clove, minced

1 teaspoon salt

1/2 cup parmesan cheese

1/2 cup ricotta cheese

1/2 teaspoon dried thyme

1/2 teaspoon crushed red pepper

1/4 cup milk

1/4 cup shaved onion

Directions:

Lightly grease a 9x13-inch baking dish with cooking spray and preheat the oven to 350oF. In a large mixing bowl, add eggs and milk. Mix thoroughly. With a paper towel, squeeze out the excess moisture from the spinach leaves and add to the bowl of eggs. Into small pieces, break the artichoke hearts and separate the leaves. Add to the bowl of eggs. Except for the ricotta cheese, add remaining ingredients in the bowl of eggs and mix thoroughly. Pour egg mixture into the prepared dish. Evenly add dollops of ricotta cheese on top of the eggs and then pop in the oven. Bake until eggs are set and doesn't jiggle when shook, about 35 minutes. Remove from the oven and evenly divide into suggested servings. Enjoy.

Nutrition: Calories 302 Protein: 22.6g Carbs: 10.8g Fat: 18.7g

Sirloin with Sweet Bell Peppers

Preparation Time: 20 minutes

Cooking Time: 8 minutes

Servings: 4

Ingredients:

12 ounces boneless top sirloin steak, about 1-inch thick, trimmed of visible fat

1 tablespoon olive oil, divided

Sea salt

Freshly ground black pepper

1 yellow bell pepper, thinly sliced

1 red bell pepper, thinly sliced

1 orange bell pepper, thinly sliced

1 small red onion, thinly sliced

4 garlic cloves, crushed

Juice of 1 lemon

Directions:

Preheat the oven to broil.

Lightly oil the steak on both sides with 1 teaspoon of olive oil and season with salt and pepper.

Place the steak on a baking sheet.

In a large bowl, toss together the bell peppers, onion, garlic, and remaining 2 teaspoons of olive oil. Season lightly with salt and pepper. Spread the vegetables on the baking sheet around the steak.

Broil the steak and vegetables until the steak is browned and the desired doneness, turning once, about 4 minutes per side.

Remove from the oven and let the steak rest for 10 minutes. Slice thinly on the bias against the grain.

Drizzle the vegetables with lemon juice and serve.

Nutrition:
Calories: 170

Total fat: 7g

Saturated fat: 2g

Carbohydrates: 11g

Sugar: 2g

Fiber: 2g

Protein: 18g

Quinoa and Spinach Salad with Figs and Balsamic Dressing

Preparation Time: 10 minutes, plus cooling time

Cooking Time: 15 minutes

Servings: 4

Ingredients:
- ½ cup quinoa
- 1 cup water
- 6 cups chopped spinach
- 8 ripe figs, quartered
- ¼ cup sunflower seeds
- ½ cup store-bought balsamic dressing
- ½ cup crumbled goat cheese

Directions:

Rinse the quinoa under cold running water to remove its bitter flavor. In a small saucepan, combine the quinoa and water and bring to a boil over medium heat. Reduce the heat to low and simmer, uncovered, until the liquid is absorbed, 10 to 15 minutes. Transfer to a dish and refrigerate until cool.

In a large bowl, toss the spinach, cooled quinoa, figs, and sunflower seeds until well mixed. Add the dressing, toss to coat, and transfer the salad to serving plates. Top with goat cheese and serve.

Nutrition:
- Calories: 348
- Total fat: 12g
- Saturated fat: 3g
- Carbohydrates: 54g
- Sugar: 21g
- Fiber: 7g
- Protein: 11g

Greek-Style Tuna Salad in Pita

Preparation Time: 25 minutes

Cooking Time: 0 minutes

Servings: 4

Ingredients:

2 (5-ounce) cans water-packed tuna, drained

½ English cucumber, chopped

1 yellow bell pepper, chopped

¼ cup chopped oil-packed sun-dried tomatoes

2 tablespoons pitted, chopped Kalamata olives

2 tablespoons chopped fresh parsley

1 tablespoon freshly squeezed lemon juice

Sea salt

Freshly ground black pepper

4 whole-wheat pita bread rounds, halved

½ cup crumbled feta cheese

1 cup shredded Boston lettuce

Directions:

In a large bowl, stir together the tuna, cucumber, bell pepper, sun-dried tomatoes, olives, parsley, and lemon juice. Season with salt and pepper. Scoop the tuna salad into the pita halves and top them with feta cheese and lettuce. Serve.

Nutrition:

Calories: 192

Total fat: 6g

Saturated fat: 3g

Carbohydrates: 23g

Sugar: 5g

Fiber: 3g

Protein: 14g

Delicious Broccoli Tortellini Salad

Preparation Time: 10 minutes

Cooking Time: 20 to 25 minutes

Servings: 12

Ingredients:

1 cup sunflower seeds, or any of your favorite seeds

3 heads of broccoli, fresh is best!

½ cup sugar

20 ounces cheese-filled tortellini

1 onion

2 teaspoons cider vinegar

½ cup mayonnaise

1 cup raisins-optional

Directions:

Cut your broccoli into florets and chop the onion.

Follow the directions to make the cheese-filled tortellini. Once they are cooked, drain and rinse them with cold water.

In a bowl, combine your mayonnaise, sugar, and vinegar. Whisk well to give the ingredients a dressing consistency.

In a separate large bowl, toss in your seeds, onion, tortellini, raisins, and broccoli.

Pour the salad dressing into the large bowl and toss the ingredients together. You will want to ensure everything is thoroughly mixed as you'll want a taste of the salad dressing with every bite!

Nutrition:

Calories: 272

Fats: 8.1 Grams

Carbohydrates: 38.6 Grams

Protein: 5 Grams

Chicken Drums With Peach Glaze

Preparation Time: 10 minutes

Cooking Time: 25 minutes

Servings: 4

Ingredients:

  2 pounds of chicken drums, remove the skin

  15 ounce can have sliced peaches, drain the juice

  ¼ cup cider vinegar

  ½ teaspoon paprika

  ¼ teaspoon black pepper

  ¼ cup honey

  3 garlic cloves

  ¼ teaspoon sea salt

Directions:

Before you turn your oven on, make sure that one rack is 4 inches below the broiler element. Set your oven's temperature to 500 degrees Fahrenheit. Line a large baking sheet with a piece of aluminum foil.

Set a wire cooling rack on top of the foil. Spray the rack with cooking spray.

Add the honey, peaches, garlic, vinegar, salt, paprika, and pepper into a blender. Mix until smooth. Set a medium saucepan on top of your stove and set the range temperature to medium heat.

Pour the mixture into the saucepan and bring it to a boil while stirring constantly. Once the sauce is done, divide it into two small bowls and set one off to the side. With the second bowl, brush half of the mixture onto the chicken drums.

Roast the drums for 10 minutes.

Take the drums out of the oven and switch to broiler mode.

Brush the drums with the other half of the sauce from the second bowl.

Again, place the drums back into the oven and set a timer for 5 minutes.

When the timer goes off, flip the drums over and broil for another 3 to 4 minutes.

Serve the drums with the reserved sauce and enjoy!

Nutrition:

Calories: 291

Fats: 5 Grams

Carbohydrates: 33 Grams

Protein: 30 Grams

Tuna and Cheese Bake

Preparation time: 5 minutes

Cooking time: 15 minutes

Servings: 4

Ingredients:

10 ounces canned tuna, drained and flaked

4 eggs, whisked

½ cup feta cheese, shredded

1 tablespoon chives, chopped

1 tablespoon parsley, chopped

Salt and black pepper to the taste

3 teaspoons olive oil

Directions:

Grease a baking dish with the oil, add the tuna and the rest of the ingredients except the cheese, toss and bake at 370 degrees F for 15 minutes.

Sprinkle the cheese on top, leave the mix aside for 5 minutes, slice and serve for breakfast.

Nutrition:

Calories 283

Fat 14.2

Fiber 5.6

Carbs 12.1

Protein 6.4

Instant Pot Potato Salad

Preparation time: 5 minutes,

Cook Time: 10 minutes

Servings: 2

Ingredients:

6 potatoes, peeled and cubed

4 eggs

1 cup mayonnaise

1 tablespoon dill pickle juice

Salt and pepper for taste

2 cups water

¼ cup chopped onion

2 tablespoons chopped parsley

1 tablespoon muster

Directions:

Take your steamer basket and put it in pressure cooker pot.

Add the water, potatoes, and eggs, and then cook on high pressure for 4 minutes. When finished, pull the eggs out and let them cool in cold water. Add the other ingredients together, and then the cooled potatoes and mix it in. you can then dice the eggs and put it in the salad, and then add salt and pepper for taste. Let it chill for an hour if you want that.

Nutrition:

Calories: 230,

Fat: 9 g

Carbs: 22gNet

Carbs: 15 g

Protein: 12 g

Fiber: 7 g.

Sodium 117%

North African Chicken Apricot Tagine

Preparation Time: 10 minutes

Cooking Time: 50 minutes

Servings: 4

Ingredients:

2 tablespoons olive oil, divided

1-pound boneless skinless chicken breast, cut into 1-inch chunks

½ sweet onion, chopped

1 tablespoon minced garlic

2 teaspoons peeled grated fresh ginger

2 cups cauliflower florets

2 carrots, cut in half lengthwise and sliced

1 (15-ounce) can low-sodium diced tomatoes

¼ cup chopped dried apricots

1 teaspoon ground cumin

½ teaspoon ground cinnamon

Sea salt

Directions:

Preheat the oven to 400°F. In a large ovenproof skillet, heat 1 tablespoon of olive oil. Brown the chicken until golden, about 10 minutes total. Transfer to a plate and set aside. Add the remaining 1 tablespoon of olive oil and sauté the onion, garlic, and ginger until softened, about 3 minutes. Add the cauliflower and carrots and sauté for 5 minutes more. Stir in the chicken, tomatoes and their juices, apricots, cumin, and cinnamon. Cover and braise in the oven until the vegetables are tender and the chicken is cooked through, 20 to 25 minutes. Season with salt and serve.

Nutrition: Calories: 252 Total fat: 9g Saturated fat: 1g Carbohydrates: 17g Sugar: 10g Fiber: 4g Protein: 28g

Oven-Roasted Puttanesca with Ground Beef

Preparation Time: 10 minutes

Cooking Time: 35 minutes

Servings: 4

Ingredients:

6 large tomatoes (about 2 pounds), cut into wedges

1 sweet onion, coarsely chopped

½ cup chopped sun-dried tomatoes

4 garlic cloves, thinly sliced

2 tablespoons olive oil, divided

8 ounces whole-grain fettucine

8 ounces extra-lean ground beef

½ cup pitted, halved Kalamata olives

¼ cup shredded fresh basil

Pinch red pepper flakes

Sea salt

Freshly ground black pepper

2 tablespoons grated Parmesan cheese

Directions:

Preheat the oven to 425°F and line a baking sheet with aluminum foil.

In a medium bowl, combine the tomatoes, onion, sun-dried tomatoes, garlic, and 1 tablespoon of olive oil and toss well. Transfer the tomato mixture to the baking sheet and roast in the oven until very tender, about 30 minutes.

While the vegetables are roasting, bring a large pot of water to a boil and cook the pasta according to package instructions until al dente. Drain.

While the pasta is cooking, in a large saucepan, add the remaining 1 tablespoon of olive oil and heat over medium-high heat. Brown the ground beef, about 10 minutes. Remove any oil from the pot with a spoon and discard.

Add the roasted vegetables to the saucepan along with the olives, basil, and red pepper flakes and stir to combine well, breaking up any larger chunks of vegetables.

Stir in the pasta. Season with salt and pepper and serve topped with Parmesan cheese.

Nutrition:

Calories: 433

Total fat: 15g

Saturated fat: 3g

Carbohydrates: 56g

Sugar: 13g

Fiber: 7g

Protein: 23g

Balsamic-Basted Beef Kebabs with Barley and Spinach Risotto

Preparation Time: 15 minutes plus marinating time

Cooking Time: 55 minutes

Servings: 4

Ingredients:

¼ cup olive oil, divided

2 tablespoons balsamic vinegar

2 teaspoons Dijon mustard

1-pound beef top sirloin steak, cut into 1-inch cubes

½ sweet onion, finely chopped

1 red bell pepper, chopped

2 teaspoons minced garlic

1 cup pearled barley, rinsed

3 cups low-sodium chicken stock

4 cups chopped spinach

2 tablespoons pine nuts

1 tablespoon chopped fresh thyme

Sea salt

Directions:

In a large bowl, stir together 3 tablespoons of olive oil, balsamic vinegar, and mustard until blended. Add the beef to the bowl, toss to coat, cover, and refrigerate for 30 minutes. Soak bamboo skewers in warm water.

While the meat is marinating, in a large saucepan, heat the remaining 1 tablespoon of olive oil over medium-high heat. Sauté the onion, bell pepper, and garlic until softened, about 4 minutes.

Stir in the barley and chicken stock and bring to a boil. Reduce the heat to low, cover, and simmer until the barley is tender and the liquid is absorbed, about 40 minutes.

Remove from the heat and stir in the spinach, pine nuts, and thyme. Season with salt.

Preheat a grill to medium high.

Thread the beef onto the soaked wooden skewers, leaving space between each chunk.

Grill the skewers until the beef reaches desired doneness, turning occasionally, about 10 minutes total for medium. Serve the beef skewers on the barley risotto.

Nutrition:

Calories: 445

Total fat: 15g

Saturated fat: 1g

Carbohydrates: 45g

Sugar: 3g

Fiber: 10g

Protein: 33g

Spinach and Beans Mediterranean Style Salad

Preparation Time: 5 minutes

Cooking Time: 30 minutes

Servings: 4

Ingredients:

15 ounces drained and rinsed cannellini beans

14 ounces drained, rinsed, and quartered artichoke hearts

6 ounces or 8 cups baby spinach

14 ½ ounces undrained diced tomatoes, no salt is best

1 tablespoon olive oil and any additional if you prefer

¼ teaspoon salt

2 minced garlic cloves

1 chopped onion, small in size

¼ teaspoon pepper

⅛ teaspoon crushed red pepper flakes

2 tablespoons Worcestershire sauce

Directions:

Place a saucepan on your stovetop and turn the temperature to medium-high. Let the pan warm up for a minute before you pour in the tablespoon of oil. Continue to let the oil heat up for another minute or two. Toss in your chopped onion and stir so all the pieces are bathed in oil. Sauté the onions for 3 minutes.

Add the garlic to the saucepan. Stir and sauté the ingredients for another minute.

Combine the salt, red pepper flakes, pepper, and Worcestershire sauce. Mix well and then add the tomatoes to the pan. Stir the mixture constantly for about 5 minutes.

Add the artichoke hearts, spinach, and beans. Sauté and stir occasionally to get the taste throughout the dish. Once the spinach starts to wilt, take the salad off of the heat.

Serve and enjoy immediately to get the best taste.

Nutrition:

Calories: 187

Fats: 4 Grams

Carbohydrates: 30 Grams

Protein: 8 Grams

Lasagna

Preparation Time: 5 minutes

Cooking Time: 1 hour 15 minutes

Servings: 8

Ingredients:

Lasagna noodles, oven-ready are the best, easiest, and quickest

⅓ cup flour

2 tablespoons chives, divided and chopped

½ cup white wine

2 tablespoons olive oil

1 ½ tablespoons thyme

1 teaspoon salt

1 ¼ cups shallots, chopped

1 cup boiled water

½ cup Parmigiano-Reggiano cheese

3 cups milk, reduced fat and divided

1 tablespoon butter

⅓ cup cream cheese, less fat is the best choice

6 cloves of garlic, divided and minced

½ teaspoon ground black pepper, divided

4 ounces dried shiitake mushrooms, sliced

1-ounce dried porcini mushrooms, sliced

8 ounces cremini mushrooms, sliced

Directions:

Keeping your mushrooms separated, drain them all and return them to separate containers.

Bring 1 cup of water to a boil and cook your porcini mushrooms for a half hour.

Preheat your oven to 350 degrees Fahrenheit.

Set a large pan on your stove and turn the burner to medium-high heat.

Add your butter and let it melt.

Combine the olive oil and shallots. Stir the mixture and let it cook for 3 minutes.

Pour half of the pepper, half of the salt, and mushrooms into the pan. Allow the mixture to cook for 6 to 7 minutes.

While stirring, add half of the garlic and thyme. Continue to stir for 1 minute.

Pour the wine and turn your burner temperature to high. Let the mixture boil and watch the liquid evaporate for a couple of minutes to reduce it slightly.

Turn off the burner and remove the pan from heat.

Add the cream cheese and chives. Stir thoroughly.

Set a medium-sized skillet on medium-high heat and add 1 tablespoon of oil. Let the oil come to a simmer.

Add the last of the garlic to the pan and sauté for 30 seconds.

Pour in 2 ⅓ cup milk and the liquid from the porcini mushrooms. Stir the mixture and allow it to boil.

In a bowl, combine ¼ cup of milk and the flour. Add this mixture to the heated pan. Stir until the mixture starts to thicken.

Grease a pan and add ½ cup of sauce along with a row of noodles.

Spread half of the mushroom mixture on top of the noodles.

Repeat the process, but make sure you top the lasagna with mushrooms and cheese.

Turn your timer to 45 minutes and set the pan into the oven.

Remember to garnish the lasagna with chives before enjoying!

Nutrition:

Calories: 268

Fats: 12.6 Gram

Carbohydrates: 29 Grams

Protein: 10 Grams

Teriyaki Chicken

Preparation time: 8 minutes

Cook Time: 22 minutes

Serves: 4

Ingredients:

for Teriyaki sauce

1/3 cup low-salt soy sauce

¼ cup honey

3 tablespoons arrowroot powder or corn starch

¼ cup rice wine vinegar or apple cider vinegar

¼ teaspoon dried sherry or mirin

3 tablespoons water for sauce

For chicken and rice:

1 tablespoon toasted sesame oil or olive oil

salt and black pepper for taste

½ teaspoon minced or grated ginger

1/3 cup shredded carrots

1 cup water

1/3 cup shelled edamame beans, thawed out

chopped green onions

1 medium boneless, skinless chicken breast

2 cloves minced garlic

¼ cup chopped red bell peppers

2 cups uncooked Jasmine rice washed, rinsed, and drained

1 cup broccoli florets

Sesame seeds to garnish

Directions:

Open instant pot and press sauté, and then whisk together the soy sauce, honey, vinegar, and mirin, and then, heat up the oil, and add the chicken, seasoning with salt and pepper, and sautéing for 2-3 minutes, until browned.

add ginger and garlic and cook for 20 seconds.

pour half the sauce into uncooked rice and one cup of water.

Cook on manual high pressure for 3 minutes, and then let it natural pressure release.

Add in the veggies and whisk the cornstarch slurry together and drizzle it over chicken and cook until veggies are tender, and sprinkle this with seeds and green onions, serving hot.

Nutrition:

Calories: 419,

Fat: 6g

Carbs: 81gNet

Carbs: 79g

Protein: 8g

Fiber: 2g

Sodium 64%

Buffalo Chicken Quinoa Bowls

Preparation time: 15 minutes

Cook Time: 15 minutes

Serves: 4

Ingredients:
   3 pounds boneless, skinless chicken breasts
   2 tablespoons olive oil
   2 tablespoons hot sauce
   2 tablespoons honey
   4 tablespoons butter or ghee
   1 cup buffalo wing sauce
   4 cloves minced garlic
   1 cup chopped green onions
   For the Quinoa bowls
   1 cup uncooked quinoa
   1 sliced cucumber
   2 chopped heads of lettuce
   2.5 cups water
   1 cup shredded carrots
   1 sliced avocado
   10 oz cherry tomatoes
   Ranch dressing or another dressing to serve

Directions:

For the chicken, add the breasts, oil, butter or ghee, band everything else to the instant pot, cooking on manual high for 6 minutes.

Let it natural pressure release, and from there, let it cool for 5 minutes before you shred it carefully.

For the quinoa bowls, add the quinoa to the instant pot, and cook it for about 5 minutes, and then let it sit for 5 minutes then fluff.

Mix everything together, with the quinoa first, then the buffalo chicken, and then the rest.

Nutrition:

Calories: 826 with fixings

Fat: 30g

Carbs: 60gNet

Carbs: 48g

Protein: 72g

Fiber: 12g

Sodium 76%

WEEK 2
BREAKFAST

Congratulations, you made it through Week 1! Take some time to reflect on what worked and what didn't and consider how you can use this experience to ensure Week 2 goes smoothly and successfully.

Now is the time to add more exercise if you started on the lower end of the recommendations. If you're finding it hard to drink all the water that's recommended, add lemon or cucumber slices to your water for flavor, or try some herbal teas or seltzer. Even water-based fruits and vegetables count (see here). If you stumbled, don't be hard on yourself—remember, you are creating new habits, and this takes time.

This week should be easier, though, because you have the first week under your belt and are, hopefully, becoming more familiar with journaling and tracking. Glance back at your first week's work and pat yourself on the back for a job well done, as you look forward to another exciting seven days—and enticing new foods!

WEEK 2	BREAKFAST	LUNCH	DINNER
MONDAY	Brekky Egg-potato Hash	Veggie Hummus Sandwich	Chicken Skillet
TUESDAY	Paleo Almond Banana Pancakes	Spicy Potato Salad	Lemon Faro Bowl
WEDNESDAY	Banana-Coconut Breakfast	Tomato and Halloumi Platter	Avgolemono Soup
THURSDAY	Sweet Potato Oats Waffles	Flatbread With Roasted Vegetables	Chicken Stuffed Peppers
FRIDAY	Cheese and Cauliflower Frittata With Peppers	Bean Lettuce Wraps	Salmon Skillet Dinner
SATURDAY	Sunny-Side Up Baked Eggs with Swiss Chard, Feta, and Basil	Tuscan Bean Soup with Kale	Shrimp Fra Diavolo
SUNDAY	Almond Butter Banana Chocolate Smoothie	Cucumbers with Feta, Mint, and Sumac	Crispy Mediterranean Chicken Thighs

Brekky Egg-potato Hash

Preparation Time: 25 minutes

Cooking Time: 25 minutes

Servings: 2

Ingredients:

1 zucchini, diced

1/2 cup chicken broth

½ pound cooked chicken

1 tablespoon olive oil

4 ounces shrimp

Salt and ground black pepper to taste

1 large sweet potato, diced

2 eggs

1/4 teaspoon cayenne pepper

2 teaspoons garlic powder

1 cup fresh spinach (optional)

Directions:

In a skillet, add the olive oil.

Fry the shrimp, cooked chicken and sweet potato for 2 minutes.

Add the cayenne pepper, garlic powder and salt, and toss for 4 minutes. Add the zucchini and toss for another 3 minutes.

Whisk the eggs in a bowl and add to the skillet.

Season using salt and pepper. Cover with the lid. Cook for 1 minute and add the chicken broth.

Cover and cook for another 8 minutes on high heat.

Add the spinach and toss for 2 more minutes.

Serve immediately.

Nutrition:

Calories per serving: 190 Protein: 11.7g Carbs: 2.9g Fat: 12.3g

Paleo Almond Banana Pancakes

Preparation Time: 10 minutes

Cooking Time: 10 minutes

Servings: 3

Ingredients:

¼ cup almond flour

½ teaspoon ground cinnamon

3 eggs

1 banana, mashed

1 tablespoon almond butter

1 teaspoon vanilla extract

1 teaspoon olive oil

Sliced banana to serve

Directions:

Whisk the eggs in a mixing bowl until they become fluffy.

In another bowl, mash the banana using a fork and add to the egg mixture.

Add the vanilla, almond butter, cinnamon and almond flour.

Mix into a smooth batter.

Heat the olive oil in a skillet.

Add one spoonful of the batter and fry them on both sides.

Keep doing these steps until you are done with all the batter.

Add some sliced banana on top before serving.

Nutrition:

Calories per serving: 306

Protein: 14.4g

Carbs: 3.6g

Fat: 26.0g

Banana-Coconut Breakfast

Preparation Time: 5 minutes

Cooking Time: 3 minutes

Servings: 4

Ingredients:

1 ripe banana

1 cup desiccated coconut

1 cup coconut milk

3 tablespoons raisins, chopped

2 tablespoon ground flax seed

1 teaspoon vanilla

A dash of cinnamon

A dash of nutmeg

Salt to taste

Directions:

Place all ingredients in a deep pan.

Allow to simmer for 3 minutes on low heat.

Place in individual containers.

Put a label and store in the fridge.

Allow to thaw at room temperature before heating in the microwave oven.

Nutrition:

Calories per serving:279

Carbs: 25.46g

Protein: 6.4g

Fiber: 5.9g

Sweet Potato Oats Waffles

Preparation Time: 5 minutes

Cooking Time: 10 minutes

Servings: 12 waffles

Ingredients:

   1 cup of sweet potato (cooked and puréed)

   2 cups of oats

   4 eggs (2 whole and 2 egg whites)

   2 tbsp of honey

   ½ tsp of baking powder

   2 cups of almond milk

   ½ tsp of salt

   2 tbsp of honey

   2 tbsp of extra virgin olive oil (EVOO)

   Cooking spray (for the waffle grill)

   For serving: two bananas and maple (or any other type of) syrup

Directions:

Preheat your waffle grill or iron. Blend all the ingredients until they are fully puréed.

Let the batter stand for about 8-10 minutes

Apply cooking spray to the griddle or waffle iron. Pour the batter so it makes about ⅓ up for each waffle mold. Cook the waffle for about 3-4 minutes and then switch it over to the other side.

When there is no more steam coming out of the waffle, it's done.

Serve the waffles with your favorite syrup and sliced bananas. Bon appétit!

Nutrition:

   Calories: 161

   Fat: 3g

   Carbs: 26g

Cheese and Cauliflower Frittata With Peppers

Preparation Time: 5 minutes

Cooking Time: 30 minutes

Servings: 6

Ingredients:

10 eggs

1 seeded and chopped bell pepper

½ cup grated Parmigiano-Reggiano

½ cup milk, skim

½ teaspoon cayenne pepper

1-pound cauliflower, floret

½ teaspoon saffron

2 tablespoons chopped chives

Salt and black pepper as desired

Directions:

Prepare your oven by setting the temperature to 370 degrees Fahrenheit. You should also grease a skillet suitable for the oven.

In a medium-sized bowl, add the milk and eggs. Whisk them until they are frothy.

Sprinkle the grated Parmigiano-Reggiano cheese into the frothy mixture and fold the ingredients together.

Pour in the salt, saffron, cayenne pepper, and black pepper and gently stir.

Add in the chopped bell pepper and gently stir until the ingredients are fully incorporated.

Pour the egg mixture into the skillet and cook on medium heat over your stovetop for 4 minutes.

Steam the cauliflower florets in a pan. To do this, add ½ inch of water and ½ teaspoon sea salt. Pour in the cauliflower and cover for 3 to 8 minutes. Drain any extra water.

Add the cauliflower into the mixture and gently stir.

Set the skillet into the preheated oven and turn your timer to 13 minutes. Once the mixture is golden brown in the middle, remove the frittata from the oven.

Set your skillet aside for a couple of minutes so it can cool.

Slice and garnish with chives before you serve.

Nutrition:
Calories: 207
Fats: 12 Grams
Carbohydrates: 8 Grams
Protein: 17 Grams

Sunny-Side Up Baked Eggs with Swiss Chard, Feta, and Basil

Preparation Time: 15 minutes

Cooking Time: 10 to 15 minutes

Servings: 4

Ingredients:

1 tablespoon extra-virgin olive oil, divided

½ red onion, diced

½ teaspoon kosher salt

¼ teaspoon nutmeg

⅛ teaspoon freshly ground black pepper

4 cups Swiss chard, chopped

¼ cup crumbled feta cheese

4 large eggs

¼ cup fresh basil, chopped or cut into ribbons

Directions:

Preheat the oven to 375°F. Place 4 ramekins on a half sheet pan or in a baking dish and grease lightly with olive oil.

Heat the remaining olive oil in a large skillet or sauté pan over medium heat. Add the onion, salt, nutmeg, and pepper and sauté until translucent, about 3 minutes. Add the chard and cook, stirring, until wilted, about 2 minutes.

Split the mixture among the 4 ramekins. Add 1 tablespoon feta cheese to each ramekin. Crack 1 egg on top of the mixture in each ramekin. Bake for 10 to 12 minutes, or until the egg white is set.

Allow to cool for 1 to 2 minutes, then carefully transfer the eggs from the ramekins to a plate with a fork or spatula. Garnish with the basil.

Nutrition:

Calories: 140; Total fat: 10g; Saturated fat: 3.5g; Cholesterol: 195mg; Sodium: 370mg; Potassium: 250mg; Total Carbohydrates: 4g; Fiber: 4g; Sugars: 2g; Protein: 9g; Magnesium: 40mg; Calcium: 100mg

Almond Butter Banana Chocolate Smoothie

Preparation Time: 5 minutes

Cooking Time: 0 minutes

Servings: 1

Ingredients:

¾ cup almond milk

½ medium banana, preferably frozen

¼ cup frozen blueberries

1 tablespoon almond butter

1 tablespoon unsweetened cocoa powder

1 tablespoon chia seeds

Directions:

In a blender or Vitamix, add all the ingredients. Blend to combine.

Nutrition:

Calories: 300; Total fat: 16g; Saturated fat: 1g; Cholesterol: 0mg; Sodium: 125mg; Potassium: 450mg; Total Carbohydrates: 37g; Fiber: 10g; Sugars: 17g; Protein: 8g; Magnesium: 100mg; Calcium: 460mg.

WEEK 2 – LUNCH

Veggie Hummus Sandwich

Preparation Time: 10 minutes

Cooking Time: 10 minutes

Servings: 2

Ingredients:

  4 slices of whole-grain bread

  6 tbsp of hummus

  1 cup of salad greens or spinach

  ½ cup of shredded carrot

  ½ medium bell pepper halved

  ½ cup of cucumber, sliced

  ½ avocado, mashed

Directions:

Combine all the ingredients together in a small mixing bowl. Spread hummus over a piece of toast or pita bread. Pour the mixture of cucumber, carrot, bell pepper, and greens in the sandwich. Then, cut the sandwich in half or quarters and serve or put in a plastic bag ready for your lunch at work or school.

Nutrition:

  Calories: 320

  Fat: 14g

  Carbs: 40g

Spicy Potato Salad

Preparation time: 10 minutes

Cooking time: 15 minutes

Servings: 4

Ingredients:

1 and ½ pounds baby potatoes, peeled and halved

A pinch of salt and black pepper

2 tablespoons harissa paste

6 ounces Greek yogurt

Juice of 1 lemon

¼ cup red onion, chopped

¼ cup parsley, chopped

Directions:

Put the potatoes in a pot, add water to cover, add salt, bring to a boil over medium-high heat, cook for 12 minutes, drain and transfer them to a bowl.

Add the harissa and the rest of the ingredients, toss and serve for lunch.

Nutrition:

Calories 354

Fat 19.2

Fiber 4.5

Carbs 24.7

Protein 11.2

Tomato and Halloumi Platter

Preparation time: 5 minutes

Cooking time: 4 minutes

Servings: 4

Ingredients:

1-pound tomatoes, sliced

½ pound halloumi, cut into 4 slices

2 tablespoons parsley, chopped

1 tablespoon basil, chopped

2 tablespoons olive oil

A pinch of salt and black pepper

Juice of 1 lemon

Directions:

Brush the halloumi slices with half of the oil, put them on your preheated grill and cook over medium-high heat and cook for 2 minutes on each side.

Arrange the tomato slices on a platter, season with salt and pepper, drizzle the lemon juice and the rest of the oil all over, top with the halloumi slices, sprinkle the herbs on top and serve for lunch.

Nutrition:

Calories 181

Fat 7.3

Fiber 1.4

Carbs 4.6

Protein 1.1

Flatbread With Roasted Vegetables

Preparation time: 10 minutes

Cooking time: 45 minutes

Servings: 12 slices

Ingredients:

5 ounces goat cheese

1 thinly sliced onion

2 thinly sliced tomatoes

Olive oil

¼ teaspoon pepper

⅛ teaspoon salt

16 ounces homemade or frozen pizza dough

¾ tablespoon chopped dill, fresh is better

1 thinly sliced zucchini

1 red pepper, cup into rings

Directions:

Set your oven to 400 degrees Fahrenheit.

Set the dough on a large piece of parchment paper. Use a rolling pin to roll the dough into a large rectangle.

Spread half of the goat cheese on ½ of the pizza dough.

Sprinkle half of the dill on the other half of the dough.

Fold the dough so the half with the dill is on top of the cheese.

Spread the remaining goat cheese on the pizza dough and then sprinkle the rest of the dill over the cheese.

Layer the vegetables on top in any arrangement you like.

Drizzle olive oil on top of the vegetables.

Sprinkle salt and pepper over the olive oil.

Set the piece of parchment paper on a pizza pan or baking pan and place it in the oven.

Set the timer for 22 minutes. If the edges are not a medium brown, leave the flatbread in the oven for another couple of minutes.

Remove the pizza from the oven when it is done and cut the flatbread in half lengthwise.

Slice the flatbread into 2-inch long pieces and enjoy!

Nutrition:

Calories: 170

Fats: 5 grams

Carbohydrates: 20 grams

Protein: 8 grams

Bean Lettuce Wraps

Preparation Time: 5 minutes

Cooking Time: 20 minutes

Servings: 4

Ingredients:

8 Romaine lettuce leaves

½ cup Garlic hummus or any prepared hummus

¾ cup chopped tomatoes

15 ounce can great northern beans, drained and rinsed

½ cup diced onion

1 tablespoon extra-virgin olive oil

¼ cup chopped parsley

¼ teaspoon black pepper

Directions:

Set a skillet on top of the stove range over medium heat.

In the skillet, warm the oil for a couple of minutes.

Add the onion into the oil. Stir frequently as the onion cooks for a few minutes. Combine the pepper and tomatoes and cook for another couple of minutes. Remember to stir occasionally.

Add the beans and continue to stir and cook for 2 to 3 minutes.

Turn the burner off, remove the skillet from heat, and add the parsley. Set the lettuce leaves on a flat surface and spread 1 tablespoon of hummus on each leaf.

Divide the bean mixture onto the 8 leaves. Spread the bean mixture down the center of the leaves. Fold the leaves by starting lengthwise on one side. Fold over the other side so the leaf is completely wrapped.

Serve and enjoy!

Nutrition:

Calories: 211

Fats: 8 Grams Carbohydrates: 28 Grams Protein: 10 Grams

Tuscan Bean Soup with Kale

Preparation Time: 20 minutes

Cooking Time: 25 minutes

Servings: 4

Ingredients:

2 tablespoons extra-virgin olive oil

1 onion, diced

1 carrot, diced

1 celery stalk, diced

1 teaspoon kosher salt

4 cups no-salt-added vegetable stock

1 (15-ounce) can no-salt-added or low-sodium cannellini beans, drained and rinsed

1 tablespoon fresh thyme, chopped

1 tablespoon fresh sage, chopped

1 tablespoon fresh oregano, chopped

¼ teaspoon freshly ground black pepper

1 bunch kale, stemmed and chopped

¼ cup grated Parmesan cheese (optional)

Directions:

Heat the olive oil in a large pot over medium-high heat. Add the onion, carrot, celery, and salt and sauté until translucent and slightly golden, 5 to 6 minutes.

Add the vegetable stock, beans, thyme, sage, oregano, and black pepper and bring to a boil. Turn down the heat to low, and simmer for 10 minutes. Stir in the kale and let it wilt, about 5 minutes. Sprinkle 1 tablespoon Parmesan cheese over each bowl before serving, if desired.

Nutrition:

Calories: 235; Total fat: 8g; Saturated fat: 1g; Cholesterol: 0mg; Sodium: 540mg; Potassium: 870mg; Total Carbohydrates: 35g; Fiber: 7g; Sugars: 6g; Protein: 9g; Magnesium: 105mg; Calcium: 205mg

Chicken Skillet

Preparation time: 10 minutes

Cooking time: 35 minutes

Servings: 6

Ingredients:

   6 chicken thighs, bone-in and skin-on

   Juice of 2 lemons

   1 teaspoon oregano, dried

   1 red onion, chopped

   Salt and black pepper to the taste

   1 teaspoon garlic powder

   2 garlic cloves, minced

   2 tablespoons olive oil

   2 and ½ cups chicken stock

   1 cup white rice

   1 tablespoon oregano, chopped

   1 cup green olives, pitted and sliced

   1/3 cup parsley, chopped

   ½ cup feta cheese, crumbled

Directions:

   Heat up a pan with the oil over medium heat, add the chicken thighs skin side down, cook for 4 minutes on each side and transfer to a plate.

   Add the garlic and the onion to the pan, stir and sauté for 5 minutes.

   Add the rice, salt, pepper, the stock, oregano, and lemon juice, stir, cook for 1-2 minutes more and take off the heat. Add the chicken to the pan, introduce the pan in the oven and bake at 375 degrees F for 25 minutes. Add the cheese, olives and the parsley, divide the whole mix between plates and serve for lunch.

Nutrition:

   Calories 435 - Fat 18.5 - Fiber 13.6 - Carbs 27.8 - Protein 25.6

WEEK 2
DINNER

Lemon Faro Bowl

Preparation Time: 3 Minutes

Cooking Time: 25 Minutes

Servings: 6

Ingredients:

1 Tablespoon + 2 Teaspoons Olive Oil, Divided

1 Cup Onion, Chopped

2 Cloves Garlic, Minced

1 Carrot, Shredded

2 Cups Vegetable Broth, Low Sodium

1 Cup Pearled Faro

2 Avocados, Peeled, Pitted & Sliced

1 Lemon, Small

Sea Salt to Taste

Directions:

Start by placing a saucepan over medium-high heat. Add in a tablespoon of oil and then throw in your onion once the oil is hot. Cook for about five minutes, stirring frequently to keep it from burning.

Add in your carrot and garlic. Allow it to cook for about another minute while you continue to stir. Add in your broth and faro. Allow it to come to a boil and adjust your heat to high to help. Once it boils, lower it to medium-low and cover your saucepan. Let it simmer for twenty minutes. The faro should be al dente and plump.

Pour the faro into a bowl and add in your avocado and zest. Drizzle with your remaining oil and add in your lemon wedges.

Nutrition:

Calories: 279 Protein: 7 G Fat: 14 G Carbs: 36 G Sodium: 118 mg

Avgolemono Soup

Preparation Time: 10 minutes

Cooking time: 20 minutes

Servings: 6

Ingredients:

   4 cups chicken stock

   1 cup of water

   1-pound chicken breast, shredded

   1 cup of rice, cooked

   3 egg yolks

   3 tablespoons lemon juice

   1/3 cup fresh parsley, chopped

   ½ teaspoon salt

   ¼ teaspoon ground black pepper

Directions:

   Pour water and chicken stock in the saucepan and bring to boil.

   Then pour one cup of the hot liquid in the food processor.

   Add cooked rice, egg yolks, lemon juice, and salt. Blend the mixture until smooth.

   After this, transfer the smooth rice mixture into the saucepan with remaining chicken stock liquid.

   Add shredded chicken breast, parsley, and ground black pepper.

   Boil the soup for 5 minutes more.

Nutrition:

   Calories 235

   Fat 5.6 g

   Fiber 7.6g

   Carbs 23.6 g

   Protein 4.6 g

Chicken Stuffed Peppers

Preparation time: 10 minutes

Cooking time: 0 minutes

Servings: 6

Ingredients:

1 cup Greek yogurt

2 tablespoons mustard

Salt and black pepper to the taste

1-pound rotisserie chicken meat, cubed

4 celery stalks, chopped

2 tablespoons balsamic vinegar

1 bunch scallions, sliced

¼ cup parsley, chopped

1 cucumber, sliced

3 red bell peppers, halved and deseeded

1-pint cherry tomatoes, quartered

Directions:

In a bowl, mix the chicken with the celery and the rest of the ingredients except the bell peppers and toss well.

Stuff the peppers halves with the chicken mix and serve for lunch.

Nutrition:

Calories 266

Fat 12.2

Fiber 4.5

Carbs 15.7

Protein 3.7

Salmon Skillet Dinner

Preparation Time: 10 minutes

Cooking Time: 15 to 20 minutes

Servings: 4

Ingredients:

1 teaspoon minced garlic

1 ½ cup quartered cherry tomatoes

1 tablespoon water

¼ teaspoon sea salt

1 tablespoon lemon juice, freshly squeezed is best

1 tablespoon extra-virgin olive oil

12 ounces drained and chopped roasted red peppers

1 teaspoon paprika

¼ teaspoon black pepper

1-pound salmon fillets

Directions:

Remove the skin from your salmon fillets and cut them into 8 pieces.

Turn your stove burner on medium heat and set a skillet on top.

Pour the olive oil into the skillet and let it heat up for a couple of minutes. Add the minced garlic and paprika. Sauté the ingredients for 1 minute.

Combine the roasted peppers, black pepper, tomatoes, water, and salt.

Set the heat to medium-high and bring the ingredients to a simmer. This should take 3 to 4 minutes. Remember to stir the ingredients occasionally so the tomatoes don't burn.

Add the salmon and take some of the sauce from the skillet to spoon on top of the fish so it is all covered in the mixture.

Cover the skillet and set a timer for 10 minutes. When the fish reaches 145 degrees Fahrenheit, it is cooked thoroughly.

Turn off the heat and drizzle lemon juice over the fish.

Break up the salmon into chunks and gently mix the pieces of fish with the sauce.

Serve and enjoy!

Nutrition:

Calories: 289

Fats: 13 Grams

Carbohydrates: 10 Grams

Protein: 31 Grams

Shrimp Fra Diavolo

Preparation Time: 10 minutes

Cooking Time: 10 minutes

Servings: 4

Ingredients:

2 tablespoons extra-virgin olive oil

1 onion, diced small

1 fennel bulb, cored and diced small, plus ¼ cup fronds for garnish

1 bell pepper, diced small

½ teaspoon dried oregano

½ teaspoon dried thyme

½ teaspoon kosher salt

¼ teaspoon red pepper flakes

1 (14.5-ounce) can no-salt-added diced tomatoes

1-pound shrimp, peeled and deveined

Juice of 1 lemon

Zest of 1 lemon

2 tablespoons fresh parsley, chopped, for garnish

Directions:

Heat the olive oil in a large skillet or sauté pan over medium heat. Add the onion, fennel, bell pepper, oregano, thyme, salt, and red pepper flakes and sauté until translucent, about 5 minutes.

Deglaze the pan with the juice from the canned tomatoes, scraping up any brown bits, and bring to a boil. Add the diced tomatoes and the shrimp. Lower heat to a simmer, cover, and cook until the shrimp are cooked through, about 3 minutes. Turn off the heat. Add the lemon juice and lemon zest and toss well to combine. Garnish with the parsley and the fennel fronds.

Nutrition:

Calories: 240; Total fat: 9g; Saturated fat: 1g; Cholesterol: 170mg; Sodium: 335mg; Potassium: 445mg; Total Carbohydrates: 13g; Fiber: 3g; Sugars: 7g; Protein: 25g; Magnesium: 55mg; Calcium: 105mg

Cucumbers with Feta, Mint, and Sumac

Preparation Time: 15 minutes

Cooking Time: 0 minutes

Servings: 4

Ingredients:

  1 tablespoon extra-virgin olive oil

  1 tablespoon lemon juice

  2 teaspoons ground sumac

  ½ teaspoon kosher salt

  2 hothouse or English cucumbers, diced

  ¼ cup crumbled feta cheese

  1 tablespoon fresh mint, chopped

  1 tablespoon fresh parsley, chopped

  ⅛ teaspoon red pepper flakes

Directions:

In a large bowl, whisk together the olive oil, lemon juice, sumac, and salt. Add the cucumber and feta cheese and toss well.

Transfer to a serving dish and sprinkle with the mint, parsley, and red pepper flakes.

Nutrition:

Calories: 85; Total fat: 6g; Saturated fat: 2g; Cholesterol: 8mg; Sodium: 230mg; Potassium: 295mg; Total Carbohydrates: 8g; Fiber: 1g; Sugars: 4g; Protein: 3g; Magnesium: 27mg; Calcium: 80mg

Crispy Mediterranean Chicken Thighs

Preparation Time: 5 minutes

Cooking Time: 30 to 35 minutes

Servings: 6

Ingredients:

2 tablespoons extra-virgin olive oil

2 teaspoons dried rosemary

1½ teaspoons ground cumin

1½ teaspoons ground coriander

¾ teaspoon dried oregano

⅛ teaspoon salt

6 bone-in, skin-on chicken thighs (about 3 pounds)

Directions:

Preheat the oven to 450°F. Line a baking sheet with parchment paper.

Place the olive oil and spices into a large bowl and mix together, making a paste. Add the chicken and mix together until evenly coated. Place on the prepared baking sheet.

Bake for 30 to 35 minutes, or until golden brown and the chicken registers an internal temperature of 165°F.

Nutrition:

Calories: 440; Total fat: 34g; Saturated fat: 9g; Cholesterol: 172mg; Sodium: 180mg; Potassium: 395mg; Total Carbohydrates: 1g; Fiber: 0g; Sugars: 0g; Protein: 30g; Magnesium: 40mg; Calcium: 30mg

WEEK 3 – BREAKFAST

Making changes that affect your health is a process. In Week 3, as previously, you will experiment with some foods you may have never tried before. Being healthy is best achieved by eating a variety of foods and giving your body nutrients from different food groups, so be open to the possibilities. As you continue to follow the plan this week, you may notice your skin has a new glow, you are sleeping better, and you have more energy. Get used to it—these are some of the many rewards of your new lifestyle! As you begin to feel more energized, it's a great invitation to add more reps or weight in your workouts. Remember, it's not just about what the scale says. It's also about how you feel as you become stronger and healthier.

WEEK 3	BREAKFAST	LUNCH	DINNER
MONDAY	Berry Baked Oatmeal	Italian White Bean Salad with Bell Peppers	Harissa Yogurt Chicken Thighs
TUESDAY	Egg in a "Pepper Hole" with Avocado	Wild Rice Salad with Chickpeas and Pickled Radish	Mediterranean Stuffed Chicken Breasts
WEDNESDAY	Edamame & Sweet Pea Hummus	Romesco Poached Chicken	Polenta with Sautéed Chard and Fried Eggs
THURSDAY	Oatmeal With Yogurt & Egg	Terrific Tilapia	Shrimp Mix
FRIDAY	Mushroom Spinach Omelet	Creamy Salmon Soup	Chicken and Barley
SATURDAY	Lentils and Cheddar Frittata	Healthy Mediterranean White Fish	Southwest Tofu Scramble
SUNDAY	Blueberry Scones	White Bean Soup	Mediterranean Tuna with Couscous and Pepperoncini

Berry Baked Oatmeal

Preparation Time: 10 minutes

Cooking Time: 45 to 50 minutes

Servings: 8

Ingredients:

2 cups gluten-free rolled oats

2 cups (10-ounce bag) frozen mixed berries (blueberries and raspberries work best)

2 cups plain, unsweetened almond milk

1 cup plain Greek yogurt

¼ cup maple syrup

2 tablespoons extra-virgin olive oil

2 teaspoons ground cinnamon

1 teaspoon baking powder

1 teaspoon vanilla extract

½ teaspoon kosher salt

¼ teaspoon ground nutmeg

⅛ teaspoon ground cloves

Directions:

Preheat the oven to 375°F.

Mix all the ingredients together in a large bowl. Pour into a 9-by-13-inch baking dish. Bake for 45 to 50 minutes, or until golden brown.

Nutrition:

Calories: 180; Total fat: 6g; Saturated fat: 1g; Cholesterol: 0mg; Sodium: 180mg; Potassium: 50mg; Total Carbohydrates: 28g; Fiber: 4g; Sugars: 11g; Protein: 6g; Magnesium: 4mg; Calcium: 180mg

Egg in a "Pepper Hole" with Avocado

Preparation Time: 15 minutes

Cooking Time: 5 minutes

Servings: 4

Ingredients:

4 bell peppers, any color

1 tablespoon extra-virgin olive oil

8 large eggs

¾ teaspoon kosher salt, divided

¼ teaspoon freshly ground black pepper, divided

1 avocado, peeled, pitted, and diced

¼ cup red onion, diced

¼ cup fresh basil, chopped

Juice of ½ lime

Directions:

Stem and seed the bell peppers. Cut 2 (2-inch-thick) rings from each pepper. Chop the remaining bell pepper into small dice and set aside.

Heat the olive oil in a large skillet over medium heat. Add 4 bell pepper rings, then crack 1 egg in the middle of each ring. Season with ¼ teaspoon of the salt and ⅛ teaspoon of the black pepper. Cook until the egg whites are mostly set but the yolks are still runny, 2 to 3 minutes. Gently flip and cook 1 additional minute for over easy. Move the egg–bell pepper rings to a platter or onto plates and repeat with the remaining 4 bell pepper rings.

In a medium bowl, combine the avocado, onion, basil, lime juice, reserved diced bell pepper, the remaining ¼ teaspoon kosher salt, and the remaining ⅛ teaspoon black pepper. Divide among the 4 plates.

Nutrition:

Calories: 270; Total fat: 19g; Saturated fat: 4g; Cholesterol: 370mg; Sodium: 360mg; Potassium: 590mg; Total Carbohydrates: 12g; Fiber: 5g; Sugars: 6g; Protein: 15g; Magnesium: 38mg; Calcium: 75mg

Edamame & Sweet Pea Hummus

Preparation Time: 5 minutes

Cooking Time: 2 minutes

Servings: 2

Ingredients:

½ c. edamame

½ c. peas

2 tbsps. Tahini

1 minced garlic clove

2 tbsps. chopped mint

3 tbsps. olive oil

2 wheat tortillas

2 eggs

Directions:

Blend the first 5 ingredients and 1 Tbsp. of olive oil in a food processor. Spread evenly over the wheat tortillas.

Coat pan with remaining olive oil and cook the eggs. When ready, put one egg on each tortilla.

Nutrition:

Carbs 35g

Fat 30g

Protein 20g

Calories 460

Oatmeal With Yogurt & Egg

Preparation Time: 5 minutes

Cooking Time: 2 minutes

Servings: 1

Ingredients:

⅓ c. oats

⅓ c. low-fat milk

1 egg

¼ tsp. cinnamon

¼ c. yogurt

¼ c. slashed apple

Salt

Sugar

Directions:

Blend the milk and egg. Mix in all ingredients except yogurt and apple.

Microwave until the liquid is evaporated, (for about 2 minutes).

Spread yogurt and apples on top of oatmeal.

Nutrition:

Calories 320

Carbs 46g

Fat 9g

Protein 17g

Mushroom Spinach Omelet

Preparation Time: 5 minutes

Cooking Time: 15 minutes

Servings: 2

Ingredients:

2 tbsp of olive oil

½ cup of sliced red onion

3 cups of fresh spinach

10 baby Bella mushrooms

1 oz. cream cheese

PAM cooking spray

2 egg whites

1 whole egg

green onions

Directions:

Bring a medium-sized skillet to medium heat. Drizzle olive oil and add red onions to skillet. Sauté for 3 minutes until the onions are cooked. Combine with mushrooms and sauté the mushrooms until they are brown. This will take about 4 minutes.

Now, add spinach. Sauté until spinach wilts, after about 3 minutes. Then, add salt and pepper for the taste. Let it stand.

Bring a small skillet to medium heat. Spray PAM on it.

Add an egg and two egg whites to a small bowl and whisk them together. Add the eggs to the small skillet and then let it stand for about 30 seconds to one minute. Run the edges of your spatula around the edges as they cook. Continue to do this for a few minutes.

Now add the mushroom spinach to the omelet side and then fold the omelet over it to make it cooked. Cook for about 40 seconds and then plate the omelet. Add green onions for garnish.

Nutrition: Calories: 412

Fat: 29g Carbs: 18g

Lentils and Cheddar Frittata

Preparation Time: 10 minutes

Cooking Time: 5 minutes

Servings: 4

Ingredients:

1 red onion, chopped

2 tablespoons olive oil

1 cup sweet potatoes, boiled and chopped

¾ cup ham, chopped

4 eggs, whisked

¾ cup lentils, cooked

2 tablespoons Greek yogurt

Salt and black pepper to the taste

½ cup cherry tomatoes, halved

¾ cup cheddar cheese, grated

Directions:

Heat up a pan with the oil over medium heat, add the onion, stir and sauté for 2 minutes.

Add the rest of the ingredients except the eggs and the cheese, toss and cook for 3 minutes more.

Add the eggs, sprinkle the cheese on top, cover the pan and cook for 10 minutes more.

Slice the frittata, divide between plates and serve.

Nutrition:

Calories 274

Fat 17.3

Fiber 3.5

Carbs 8.9

Protein 11.4

Blueberry Scones

Preparation Time: 15 minutes

Cooking Time: 15 minutes

Servings: 32 Scones

Ingredients:

4 cups of almond flour (not almond meal)

1 cup of baking soda

1 teaspoon of Celtic sea salt

1 cup of dried blueberries

½ cup of sunflower seeds

½ cup of raw sesame seeds

½ cup of pistachios, coarsely chopped

2 large eggs - Use large eggs, otherwise the dough will not hold together properly.

4 tbsp of nectar or honey

Directions:

In a mixing bowl, combine almond flour, sea salt, and baking soda.

Mix in the dried blueberries, seeds, and pistachios.

In a small mixing bowl, combine the large egg with the agave.

Combine the wet ingredients so they dry. Use your hands so you can form the dough. Make 6x6 squares that are about ½-inch thick.

Cut the dough so that it makes 32 squares.

Put the dough on two baking sheets (16 squares each) and put in the oven Bake at 350 degrees Fahrenheit with a parchment-paper-lined pan for 10-12 minutes. Serve.

Nutrition:

Calories: 380

Fat: 17g

Carbs: 45g

WEEK 3
LUNCH

Italian White Bean Salad with Bell Peppers

Preparation Time: 4 minutes

Cooking Time: 15 minutes

Servings: 4

Ingredients:

2 tablespoons extra-virgin olive oil

2 tablespoons white wine vinegar

½ shallot, minced

½ teaspoon kosher salt

¼ teaspoon freshly ground black pepper

3 cups cooked cannellini beans, or 2 (15-ounce) cans no-salt-added or low-sodium cannellini beans, drained and rinsed

2 celery stalks, diced

½ red bell pepper, diced

¼ cup fresh parsley, chopped

¼ cup fresh mint, chopped

Directions:

In a large bowl, whisk together the olive oil, vinegar, shallot, salt, and black pepper.

Add the beans, celery, red bell pepper, parsley, and mint; mix well.

Nutrition:

Calories: 300; Total fat: 8g; Saturated fat: 1g; Cholesterol: 0mg; Sodium: 175mg; Potassium: 1100mg; Total Carbohydrates: 46g; Fiber: 11g; Sugars: 3g; Protein: 15g; Magnesium: 115mg; Calcium: 175mg

Wild Rice Salad with Chickpeas and Pickled Radish

Preparation Time: 20 minutes

Cooking Time: 45 minutes

Servings: 4

Ingredients:

FOR THE RICE

1 cup water

4 ounces (⅔ cup) wild rice

¼ teaspoon kosher salt

FOR THE PICKLED RADISH

1 bunch radishes (6 to 8 small), sliced thin

½ cup white wine vinegar

½ teaspoon kosher salt

FOR THE DRESSING

2 tablespoons extra-virgin olive oil

2 tablespoons white wine vinegar

½ teaspoon pure maple syrup

½ teaspoon kosher salt

¼ teaspoon freshly ground black pepper

FOR THE SALAD

1 (15-ounce) can no-salt-added or low-sodium chickpeas, rinsed and drained

1 bulb fennel, diced

¼ cup walnuts, chopped and toasted

¼ cup crumbled feta cheese

¼ cup currants

2 tablespoons fresh dill, chopped

Directions:

TO MAKE THE RICE

Bring the water, rice, and salt to a boil in a medium saucepan. Cover reduce the heat, and simmer for 45 minutes.

TO MAKE THE PICKLED RADISH

In a medium bowl, combine the radishes, vinegar, and salt. Let sit for 15 to 30 minutes.

TO MAKE THE DRESSING

In a large bowl, whisk together the olive oil, vinegar, maple syrup, salt, and black pepper.

TO MAKE THE SALAD

1 While still warm, add the rice to the bowl with the dressing and mix well.

2 Add the chickpeas, fennel, walnuts, feta, currants, and dill. Mix well.

3 Garnish with the pickled radishes before serving.

Nutrition:

Calories: 310; Total fat: 16g; Saturated fat: 3g; Cholesterol: 8mg; Sodium: 400mg; Potassium: 415mg; Total Carbohydrates: 36g; Fiber: 7g; Sugars: 11g; Protein: 10g; Magnesium: 70mg; Calcium: 110mg

Romesco Poached Chicken

Preparation Time: 10 minutes

Cooking Time: 20 minutes

Servings: 6

Ingredients:

1½ pounds boneless, skinless chicken breasts, cut into 6 pieces

1 carrot, halved

1 celery stalk, halved

½ onion halved

2 garlic cloves, smashed

3 sprigs fresh thyme or rosemary

1 cup Romesco Dip

2 tablespoons chopped fresh flat-leaf (Italian) parsley

¼ teaspoon freshly ground black pepper

Directions:

Put the chicken in a medium saucepan. Fill with water until there's about one inch of liquid above the chicken. Add the carrot, celery, onion, garlic, and thyme. Cover and bring it to a boil. Reduce the heat to low (keeping it covered), and cook for 12 to 15 minutes, or until the internal temperature of the chicken measures 165°F on a meat thermometer and any juices run clear.

Remove the chicken from the water and let sit for 5 minutes.

When you're ready to serve, spread ¾ cup of romesco dip on the bottom of a serving platter. Arrange the chicken breasts on top, and drizzle with the remaining romesco dip. Sprinkle the tops with parsley and pepper.

Nutrition:

Calories: 237 Total Fat: 11g

Saturated Fat: 1g Cholesterol: 65mg Sodium: 336mg

Total Carbohydrates: 8g Fiber: 4g Protein: 28g

Terrific Tilapia

Preparation Time: 15 minutes

Cooking Time: 15 minutes

Servings: 2

Ingredients:

2 tilapia fillets

3 tbsp of sun-dried tomatoes, drained and chopped

1 tbsp of capers, drained

1 tbsp of oil from the sun-dried tomato jar

2 tbsp of Kalamata olives, pitted and slice

1 tbsp of lemon juice

Directions:

Heat the oven to 375 degrees Fahrenheit. Toss the tomatoes, capers, and olives and then set aside. Put the tilapia in a baking dish and pour on some oil and lemon juice.

Bake for 12-15 minutes in the oven until the fish makes flakes when pinched with a fork. Make sure to not overcook the fish or it may become dry. After the fish is finished, pour the tomato sauce on top and then serve immediately. Refrigerate the leftovers in a microwaveable container.

Nutrition:

Calories: 248

Fat: 3g

Carbs: 11g

Creamy Salmon Soup

Preparation time: 10 minutes

Cooking time: 15 minutes

Servings: 6

Ingredients:

2 tablespoon olive oil

1 red onion, chopped

Salt and white pepper to the taste

3 gold potatoes, peeled and cubed

2 carrots, chopped

4 cups fish stock

4 ounces salmon fillets, boneless and cubed

½ cup heavy cream

1 tablespoon dill, chopped

Directions:

Heat up a pan with the oil over medium heat, add the onion, and sauté for 5 minutes.

Add the rest of the ingredients expect the cream, salmon and the dill, bring to a simmer and cook for 5-6 minutes more.

Add the salmon, cream and the dill, simmer for 5 minutes more, divide into bowls and serve.

Nutrition:

Calories 214

Fat 16.3

Fiber 1.5

Carbs 6.4

Protein 11.8

Healthy Mediterranean White Fish

Preparation Time: 10 minutes

Cooking Time: 20 minutes

Servings: 8

Ingredients:

2 tbsp of extra virgin olive oil (EVOO)

4-6 cloves of garlic

½ cup of fresh basil

salt and pepper

2 cans of tomatoes (28 oz. each)

8 fillets of white fish

2 tbsp of capers

8 oz. of Kalamata olives

2 lemons, thinly sliced

Directions:

Preheat the oven to 375 degrees Fahrenheit.

Sauté your garlic in a frying pan until fragrant. Then, toss in some crushed tomatoes, salt and pepper, and basil. With a cast-iron pan, you can put it in the oven, which can make the flavors mix better.

Coat your ovenproof dish/pan with your tomato sauce. Put the fish on top of the sauce and then spread some sliced lemons on the fish. Sprinkle some olives and capers on the fish and tomato sauce. Then, add some EVOO before baking in the oven.

Bake the fish uncovered for about 25-30 minutes or until the fish form flakes in your fork.

Optional garnish of basil on the side. Bon appétit!

Nutrition:

Calories: 225

Fat: 4g

Carbs: 17g

White Bean Soup

Preparation Time: 9-10 minutes

Cooking Time: 24-25 minutes

Servings: 3

Ingredients:

½ tbs olive oil

½ large onion

1 garlic clove minced

½ of a large carrot

½ celery stick

½ tsp of dried thyme

3 cups of vegetable broth

¼ tsp of oregano

¼ tsp of black pepper

½ tsp of kosher salt

2 15 oz. canned white beans, drained and rinsed

1 cup of baby spinach

Parmesan-Reggiano cheese, for serving

Fresh parsley, for serving

Directions:

In a large soup pot or saucepan, put the olive oil on high heat. Sauté onions and garlic and then add carrots, oregano, salt and pepper, thyme, and continue cooking for about 3 minutes. Add vegetable broth and beans. Bring everything to a boil and then turn down the heat and allow it to simmer for 15-20 minutes and let all the flavors combine.

Add the spinach and continue simmering until the spinach is wilted, after about 3 minutes. Take the pan off the heat and then pour parsley and Parmesan-Reggiano cheese over it. Serve immediately. Store the leftovers in a microwaveable container for reheating later.

Nutrition:

Calories: 250 Fat: 3g Carbs: 55g

Harissa Yogurt Chicken Thighs

Preparation Time: 5 minutes, plus 15 minutes to marinate

Cooking Time: 25 minutes

Servings: 4

Ingredients:
- ½ cup plain Greek yogurt
- 2 tablespoons harissa
- 1 tablespoon lemon juice
- ½ teaspoon kosher salt
- ¼ teaspoon freshly ground black pepper
- 1½ pounds boneless, skinless chicken thighs

Directions:

In a bowl, combine the yogurt, harissa, lemon juice, salt, and black pepper. Add the chicken and mix together. Marinate for at least 15 minutes, and up to 4 hours in the refrigerator.

Preheat the oven to 425°F. Line a baking sheet with parchment paper or foil. Remove the chicken thighs from the marinade and arrange in a single layer on the baking sheet. Roast for 20 minutes, turning the chicken over halfway.

Change the oven temperature to broil. Broil the chicken until golden brown in spots, 2 to 3 minutes.

Nutrition:

Calories: 190; Total fat: 10g; Saturated fat: 2g; Cholesterol: 107mg; Sodium: 230mg; Potassium: 300mg; Total Carbohydrates: 1g; Fiber: 0g; Sugars: 1g; Protein: 24g; Magnesium: 28mg; Calcium: 24mg

Mediterranean Stuffed Chicken Breasts

Preparation Time: 10 minutes

Cooking Time: 15 minutes

Servings: 8

Ingredients:

8 oz. chicken breasts

1 Large red bell pepper

2 tbsps. chopped Kalamata olives

¼ c. crumbled feta cheese

1 tbsp. fresh basil

Directions:

Begin by preheating your broiler. On a chopping block, start cutting your bell pepper in half, lengthwise and get rid of all of the membrane and seeds. On a baking sheet, place the pepper halves skin side up and flatten them with your hand. Place the peppers into the oven and broil for about 15 minutes or until they have blackened. Once they are prepared, place the peppers into a zip lock bag and allow them to sit for about 15 minutes. When the time has passed, peel the peppers and chop them. When this is done, place a pan on your grill over medium-high heat and place your cheese, olives, basil, and bell pepper. With your chicken, you will want to slice a horizontal slit through the thickest part of the chicken to form some sort of a pocket. Once this is done, place the pepper mixture into each of your chicken breasts and then close the pocket with a wooden toothpick. Sprinkle pepper and salt over the chicken and place the chicken on a grill rack. Grill each side for about 6 minutes on both sides or until it is thoroughly cooked.

Once cooked, allow the chicken to stand for about 10 minutes. Your meal is ready to be served once it is cooled!

Nutrition:

Calories 210 Fat - 5.9g - Protein 35.2g - Carbs 1.8g

Polenta with Sautéed Chard and Fried Eggs

Preparation Time: 5 minutes

Cooking Time: 20 minutes

Servings: 4

Ingredients:

FOR THE POLENTA

2½ cups water

½ teaspoon kosher salt

¾ cups whole-grain cornmeal

¼ teaspoon freshly ground black pepper

2 tablespoons grated Parmesan cheese

FOR THE CHARD

1 tablespoon extra-virgin olive oil

1 bunch (about 6 ounces) Swiss chard, leaves and stems chopped and separated

2 garlic cloves, sliced

¼ teaspoon kosher salt

⅛ teaspoon freshly ground black pepper

Lemon juice (optional)

FOR THE EGGS

1 tablespoon extra-virgin olive oil

4 large eggs

Directions:

TO MAKE THE POLENTA

1 Bring the water and salt to a boil in a medium saucepan over high heat. Slowly add the cornmeal, whisking constantly.

2 Decrease the heat to low, cover, and cook for 10 to 15 minutes, stirring often to avoid lumps. Stir in the pepper and Parmesan and divide among 4 bowls.

TO MAKE THE CHARD

3 Heat the oil in a large skillet over medium heat. Add the chard

stems, garlic, salt, and pepper; sauté for 2 minutes. Add the chard leaves and cook until wilted, about 3 to 5 minutes.

4 Add a spritz of lemon juice (if desired), toss together, and divide evenly on top of the polenta.

TO MAKE THE EGGS

5 Heat the oil in the same large skillet over medium-high heat. Crack each egg into the skillet, taking care not to crowd the skillet and leaving space between the eggs. Cook until the whites are set and golden around the edges, about 2 to 3 minutes.

6 Serve sunny-side up or flip the eggs over carefully and cook 1 minute longer for over easy. Place one egg on top of the polenta and chard in each bowl.

Nutrition:

Calories: 310; Total fat: 18g; Saturated fat: 5g; Cholesterol: 375mg; Sodium: 500mg; Potassium: 385mg; Total Carbohydrates: 21g; Fiber: 2g; Sugars: 1g; Protein: 17g; Magnesium: 80mg; Calcium: 120mg

Shrimp Mix

Preparation Time: 10 minutes

Cooking Time: 10 minutes

Servings: 4

Ingredients:

1 and ½ pounds shrimp, peeled and deveined

1 tablespoon olive oil

1 teaspoon sesame seeds

24 ounces broccoli florets

1 green onion, chopped

1 tablespoon balsamic vinegar

2 garlic cloves, minced

1 tablespoon ginger, grated

Directions:

In a bowl, mix oil with vinegar, garlic and ginger and whisk.

Transfer this to a pan, heat up over medium heat, add shrimp, stir and cook for 3 minutes.

Add broccoli, stir, cook for 4 minutes more,

Add sesame seeds and green onions, toss, divide everything between plates and serve.

Nutrition:

Calories: 265

Protein: 20 G

Fat: 2G

Carbs: 10 G

Chicken and Barley

Preparation time: 15 minutes,

Cook Time: 35 minutes

Servings: 4

Ingredients:

    6 oz. Barley

    1-pound chicken thighs

    5 chopped carrots

    12 oz, water

    5 oz. Peas

    3 chopped yellow onions

    6 oz. Low-

    Sodium veggie stock

    Black pepper for taste

Directions:

Within the instant pot, mix the stock with the barley and water, and cook on highs for 20 minutes.

Add in onions, carrots, peas, and chicken, and then cook on high once again, natural pressure release.

Add more black pepper for taste, and then serve!

Nutrition:

    Calories: 261,

    Fat: 7g

    Carbs: 18gNet

    Carbs: 10g

    Protein: 7g

    Fiber: 8g

    Sodium 39%

Southwest Tofu Scramble

Preparation Time: 10 minutes

Cooking Time: 20 minutes

Servings: 4

Ingredients:

Scramble with Tofu

16 oz. firm tofu

2-4 Tbsp of extra virgin olive oil (EVOO)

½ red onion (sliced)

1 red pepper (thinly sliced)

4 cups of kale

Sauce

1 tsp garlic powder

0.5 tsp turmeric (optional)

1 tsp chili powder

1 tsp sea salt

Water (to thin)

Optional ingredients:

Tex-Mex salsa

Cilantro

4 pieces of toast

Banana and orange, or other fruit

Directions:

Dry the tofu on a paper towel and then add to a cast-iron skillet for 13-14 minutes.

After the tofu is dry, mix the sauce by adding spices to a small mixing bowl and then add enough water to incorporate into the sauce.

Heat the veggies over medium heat. After they have heated, drizzle EVOO over the onion and red pepper. And then add salt to taste and stir. Cook everything until soft, after about 3-4 minutes.

Mix in kale, add more salt and pepper. Steam for 3 minutes.

Crumble the tofu into bite-sized pieces.

Add the tofu to pan and move the veggies to the other side. Sauté for 1.5-2 minutes, and then add sauce. Pour it over the tofu and slightly on the veggies.

Stir all the ingredients together and then pour over the sauce. Cook for another 6-7 minutes until the tofu becomes brown.

Serve immediately. Garnish with toast, fruit, or breakfast potatoes. To spice things up, add Tex-Mex salsa or fresh cilantro. You can also freeze the dish for up to one month and reheat on the stove or in the microwave.

Nutrition:

Calories: 212

Fat: 15.1g

Carbs: 7.1g

Mediterranean Tuna with Couscous and Pepperoncini

Preparation Time: 4 minutes

Cooking Time: 12 minutes

Servings: 8

Ingredients:

Topping

4 5-oz. cans of oil packed tuna

1 cup of sliced pepperoncini

⅔ cup of fresh parsley

2 pints of cherry tomatoes, sliced and halved

EVOO, for serving

2 lemons, quartered

Sea salt and freshly ground pepper, for taste

Couscous

2 ½ cups of couscous

1 ½ tsp of sea salt

2 cups of chicken broth or water

Directions:

Prepare the Couscous:

In a small pot, boil water or broth over medium heat. Take the pot off the heat. Add couscous and stir; cover and let sit for 10 minutes.

Make the Topping:

Now, combine the tomatoes, pepperoncini, capers, tomatoes, and parsley in a medium-sized mixing bowl. Set aside.

Add EVOO to pan with couscous and add a pinch of salt and pepper. Add the tuna mixture to the couscous.

Serve immediately and garnish with lemon.

Nutrition:

Calories: 226 Fat: 1g Carbs: 44g

WEEK 4
BREAKFAST

Congratulations again—the final week of your 28-day diet plan is here! By now you are most likely craving less sugar and fewer refined carbs. This week, you may be tempted by a coworker's birthday cake or a friend's invitation to go for ice cream but remember why you started. You committed to finishing this plan, and you are one food shop and prep away from achieving that. You will have birthday cake again—but Week 4 is especially important because it solidifies your commitment to the plan and your dedication to eating healthy. You'll continue to try new recipes and now you can mark which ones you like the best so you can make them again. Celebrate this last week by sharing your experience with a friend or family member—invite them over to try a favorite dish or two. You will also be rounding out your 28-day trial with the "personal trainer" and continuing to use your logs to track your habits.

WEEK 4	BREAKFAST	LUNCH	DINNER
MONDAY	Baked Eggs With Spinach	Rosemary Minestrone	Artichokes, Olives & Tuna Pasta
TUESDAY	Quinoa & Dried Fruit	Beefaroni Soup	Glazed Ribs
WEDNESDAY	Eggs & Hash & Cheese	Pasta with Meat Sauce	Tavern Sandwiches in Instant Pot
THURSDAY	Veggie Breakfast Bowl	Instant Pot Shredded Chicken	Tuscan Chicken Pasta
FRIDAY	Apple Peanut Butter Oatmeal	Orzo Soup with Kale	Chinese Chicken
SATURDAY	Muffin Pan Frittatas	Portobello Mushroom Pizza	Bell Peppers 'n Tomato-Chickpea Rice
SUNDAY	Mediterranean Breakfast Sandwich	Tasty Lasagna Rolls	Avocado and Turkey Mix Panini

Baked Eggs With Spinach

Preparation Time: 5 minutes

Cooking Time: 20 minutes

Servings: 4

Ingredients:

4 eggs

1 package frozen spinach

¼ c. shredded Cheddar cheese

¼ c. chunky salsa

Directions:

Preheat oven to 325°F.

Put an equal amount of spinach into 4 custard cups. Make a well in the middle by pressing down with your fingers.

Add an egg into each indentation. Spoon salsa and shredded cheese on the top.

Cook for 20 min.

Nutrition:

Calories 120

Carbs 4g

Fat 7g

Protein 10g

Quinoa & Dried Fruit

Preparation Time: 10 minutes

Cooking Time: 15 minutes

Servings: 4

Ingredients:

3 c. water

1 c. quinoa

¼ c. walnuts

8 dried apricots

4 dried figs

1 tsp. cinnamon

Directions:

In a pot, mix water and quinoa and let simmer for 15 minutes, until the water evaporates.

Chop dried fruit.

When quinoa is cooked, stir in all other ingredients.

Serve cold. Add milk, if desired.

Nutrition:

Carbs 44g

Fat 7g

Protein 13g

Calories 285

Eggs & Hash & Cheese

Preparation Time: 5 minutes

Cooking Time: 2 minutes

Servings: 1

Ingredients:

1 egg

½ c. shredded hash browns

2 tbsps. cheddar cheese

Salt

Pepper

Directions:

Grease a microwaveable bowl with olive oil spray and fill with hash browns. Microwave for 1 minute and add salt and pepper to taste.

Stir in an egg and beat well. Microwave for 45 seconds.

Sprinkle cheese over the top.

Nutrition:

Carbs 7g

Fat 14g

Protein 15g

Calories 210

Veggie Breakfast Bowl

Preparation Time: 5 minutes

Cooking Time: 2 minutes

Servings: 1

Ingredients:

   1 egg

   1 tbsp. water

   2 tbsps. shredded mozzarella cheese

   2 tbsps. diced mushrooms

   ¼ c. baby spinach

   2 tbsps. cherry tomatoes

Directions:

   Mix all ingredients excluding the cheese in a greased microwaveable bowl.

   Microwave for 1 minute or until the egg is cooked.

   Sprinkle shredded cheese over the top.

Nutrition:

   Carbs 2g

   Fat 6g

   Protein 10g

   Calories 100

Apple Peanut Butter Oatmeal

Preparation Time: 15 minutes

Cooking Time: 8 hours

Servings: 4

Ingredients:

1 c. steel-cut oats

¼ c. brown sugar

½ tsp. cinnamon

¼ c. peanut butter

1 tsp. vanilla extract

2 diced apples

Salt

Directions:

Grease a slow cooker with cooking spray.

Add all ingredients to the crockpot except apples, mix well.

Add apples to the top of the mixture and cook on low for 8 hours.

Nutrition:

Carbs 50g

Fat 11g

Protein 10g

Calories 320

Muffin Pan Frittatas

Preparation Time: 10 minutes

Cooking Time: 15 minutes

Servings: 6

Ingredients:

6 eggs

½ c. milk

1 c. cheddar cheese

¾ c. chopped zucchini

¼ c. chopped red bell pepper

2 tbsps. sliced red onion

Pepper

Directions:

Preheat oven to 350°F.

Mix the milk, eggs, and pepper. Then mix in other ingredients.

Spray cooking spray on a muffin tin and distribute the prepared mixture evenly between the cups. Bake for 15 min.

Nutrition:

Carbs 3g

Fat 10g

Protein 12g

Calories 165

Mediterranean Breakfast Sandwich

Preparation Time: 5 minutes

Cooking Time: 5 minutes

Servings: 1

Ingredients:

1 Heirloom Tomato

1 Onion

2 slices of Bread

¼ Zucchini

1 Egg

1 tbsp. Basil

Salt

Directions:

Begin by thinly slicing the onion, zucchini, tomato, and basil leaves.

Place the olive oil into the pan on medium heat and add an egg. The style of the egg is up to you.

Meanwhile, toast your bread slices in a toaster.

Place one slice of bread onto a plate and lay the egg on top.

In the pan, set the zucchini and onion and allow them to brown. This should take only a few minutes.

On the other slice of bread, layer your tomato and basil.

Once your onion and zucchini are soft, layer them on top of the tomato and basil.

Finally, layer the bread pieces on top of one another and your sandwich is complete!

Nutrition:

Calories 242

Carbs 25g

Fat 12g

Protein 13g

Rosemary Minestrone

Preparation Time: 5 minutes

Cooking time: 25 minutes

Servings: 4

Ingredients:
   2 oz celery stalk, chopped

   1 russet potato, chopped

   ½ cup butternut squash, chopped

   1 teaspoon fresh rosemary

   ½ teaspoon salt

   ½ teaspoon ground black pepper

   2 oz Parmesan, grated

   1 tablespoon butter

   ½ zucchini, chopped

   ¼ cup green beans, chopped

   2 oz whole wheat pasta

   4 cups chicken stock

   ½ teaspoon tomato paste

   ¾ cup red kidney beans, canned, drained

Directions:
In the saucepan combine together celery stalk, potato, butternut squash, rosemary, salt, ground black pepper, butter, and stir well.

Cook the vegetables for 5 minutes over the medium-low heat.

After this, add zucchini, green beans, whole wheat pasta, chicken stock, and tomato paste.

Add red kidney beans and chicken stock.

Stir the soup well and cook it for 15 minutes over the medium-high heat.

Then add Parmesan and stir minestrone.

Cook it for 2 minutes more.

Ladle minestrone in the serving bowls immediately.

Nutrition:

Calories 234

Fat 6.5

Fiber 10.1

Carbs 39.7

Protein 31.1

Beefaroni Soup

Preparation Time: 10 minutes

Cooking time: 30 minutes

Servings: 6

Ingredients:

½ cup elbow macaroni

1 teaspoon coconut oil

1/3 teaspoon minced garlic

2 oz yellow onion, diced

1 ½ cup ground beef

½ teaspoon dried oregano

½ teaspoon dried thyme

1 teaspoon salt

1 teaspoon chili flakes

3 oz Mozzarella, shredded

1 teaspoon dried basil

5 cups beef broth

1 tablespoon cream cheese

1 cup water, for cooking macaroni

Directions:

Pour water in the pan and bring it to boil.

Add elbow macaroni and cook them according to the manufacturer directions.

Then drain water from the cooked elbow macaroni.

Put coconut oil in the big pot and melt it.

Add minced garlic, yellow onion, ground beef, dried oregano, dried thyme, salt, chili flakes, and dried basil.

Cook the ingredients for 10 minutes over the medium-low heat. Stir the mixture from time to time.

Add beef broth and cream cheese. Stir the soup until it is homogenous.

Cook the soup for 10 minutes.

Then add cooked elbow macaroni and stir well.

Bring the soup to boil and remove from the heat.

Ladle the cooked soup in the serving bowls and garnish with Mozzarella.

Nutrition:

Calories 178

Fat 3.5

Fiber 6.1

Carbs 24.7

Protein 21.1

Pasta with Meat sauce

Preparation time: 10 minutes

Cook Time: 5 minutes

Servings: 4-6

Ingredients:

  2 cloves minced garlic

  1 diced red pepper

  8 oz. Dried pasta

  12 oz. Water

  1 diced small onion

  2 pounds ground meat

  1 jar pasta sauce

Directions:

  Turn instant pot to sauté setting.

  Add in onions, peppers, and meat to cook till no longer pink.

  Add pasta, pasta sauce, and water, and stir it.

  Set it for 5 minutes manual mode, and then quick release, top with cheese and parsley.

Nutrition:

  Calories: 437

  Fat: 25g

  Carbs: 30gNet

  Carbs: 26g

  Protein: 24g

  Fiber: 4g

  Sodium 6%

Instant Pot Shredded Chicken

Preparation time: 10 minutes

Cook Time: 16 minutes

Servings: 4

Ingredients:
pounds boneless, skinless chicken breasts

1 teaspoon oregano, dried

½ teaspoon salt

1 cup low-

Sodium chicken broth

½ teaspoon garlic powder

¼ teaspoon black pepper

Directions:
Put chicken within instant pot, then the broth, and rest of the ingredients.

Cook on high pressure for 16 minutes for larger breasts, and then natural pressure release for a couple minutes, but then quick release.

When finished, check the temperature, making sure it's 165 degrees.

Remove chicken, and then shred it, and stir in the broth to flavor it, and then serve in bowls.

Nutrition:
Calories: 169

Fat: 4g

Carbs: 5gNet

Carbs: 1g

Protein: 30g

Fiber: 3g

Orzo Soup with Kale

Preparation Time: 10 minutes

Cooking time: 20 minutes

Servings: 4

Ingredients:

1/3 cup orzo pasta

¼ white onion, diced

1 oz celery stalk, chopped

½ teaspoon chili flakes

½ teaspoon salt

1 garlic clove, diced

1 cup kale, chopped

½ cup tomatoes, chopped

1 carrot, chopped

½ teaspoon dried thyme

½ teaspoon dried oregano

5 cups vegetable stock

Directions:

Pour the vegetable stock in the pan and bring it to boil.

Add celery stalk and diced onion. After this, sprinkle the liquid with chili flakes and salt.

Add diced garlic, tomatoes, carrot, dried thyme, and dried oregano.

Bring the liquid to boil. Add orzo pasta and cook it for 5 minutes.

After this, add kale and cook the soup for 3 minutes more.

Remove the soup from the heat and leave it to rest with the closed lid for 10 minutes.

Nutrition:

Calories 74

Fat 6.5 Fiber 5.1 Carbs 2.7 Protein 3.1

Portobello Mushroom Pizza

Preparation Time: 12 minutes

Cooking Time: 12 minutes

Servings: 4

Ingredients:

½ teaspoon red pepper flakes

A handful of fresh basil, chopped

1 can black olives, chopped

1 medium onion, chopped

1 green pepper, chopped

¼ cup chopped roasted yellow peppers

½ cup prepared nut cheese, shredded

2 cups prepared gluten-free pizza sauce

8 Portobello mushrooms, cleaned and stems removed

Directions:

Preheat the oven toaster.

Take a baking sheet and grease it. Set aside.

Place the Portobello mushroom cap-side down and spoon 2 tablespoon of packaged pizza sauce on the underside of each cap. Add nut cheese and top with the remaining ingredients.

Broil for 12 minutes or until the toppings are wilted.

Nutrition:

Calories per Serving: 578

Carbs: 73.0g;

Protein: 24.4g

Fat: 22.4g

Tasty Lasagna Rolls

Preparation Time: 20 minutes

Cooking Time: 20 minutes

Servings: 6

Ingredients:

¼ tsp crushed red pepper

¼ tsp salt

½ cup shredded mozzarella cheese

½ cups parmesan cheese, shredded

1 14-oz package tofu, cubed

1 25-oz can of low-sodium marinara sauce

1 tbsp extra virgin olive oil

12 whole wheat lasagna noodles

2 tbsp Kalamata olives, chopped

3 cloves minced garlic

3 cups spinach, chopped

Directions:

Put enough water on a large pot and cook the lasagna noodles according to package instructions. Drain, rinse and set aside until ready to use. In a large skillet, sauté garlic over medium heat for 20 seconds. Add the tofu and spinach and cook until the spinach wilts. Transfer this mixture in a bowl and add parmesan olives, salt, red pepper and 2/3 cup of the marinara sauce. In a pan, spread a cup of marinara sauce on the bottom. To make the rolls, place noodle on a surface and spread ¼ cup of the tofu filling. Roll up and place it on the pan with the marinara sauce. Do this procedure until all lasagna noodles are rolled.

Place the pan over high heat and bring to a simmer. Reduce the heat to medium and let it cook for three more minutes. Sprinkle mozzarella cheese and let the cheese melt for two minutes. Serve hot.

Nutrition: Calories: 304 Carbs: 39.2g Protein: 23g Fat: 19.2

Artichokes, Olives & Tuna Pasta

Preparation Time: 15 Minutes

Cooking Time: 15 Minutes

Servings: 4

Ingredients:

¼ cup chopped fresh basil

¼ cup chopped green olives

¼ tsp freshly ground pepper

½ cup white wine

½ tsp salt, divided

1 10-oz package frozen artichoke hearts, thawed and squeezed dry

2 cups grape tomatoes, halved

2 tbsp lemon juice

2 tsp chopped fresh rosemary

2 tsp freshly grated lemon zest

3 cloves garlic, minced

4 tbsp extra virgin olive oil, divided

6-oz whole wheat penne pasta

8-oz tuna steak, cut into 3 pieces

Directions:

Cook penne pasta according to package instructions. Drain and set aside. Preheat grill to medium high.

In bowl, toss and mix ¼ tsp pepper, ¼ tsp salt, 1 tsp rosemary, lemon zest, 1 tbsp oil and tuna pieces.

Grill tuna for 3 minutes per side. Allow to cool and flake into bite sized pieces. On medium fire, place a large nonstick saucepan and heat 3 tbsp oil.

Sauté remaining rosemary, garlic olives, and artichoke hearts for 4 minutes

Add wine and tomatoes, bring to a boil and cook for 3 minutes while stirring once in a while.

Add remaining salt, lemon juice, tuna pieces and pasta. Cook until heated through.

To serve, garnish with basil and enjoy.

Nutrition:

Calories per Serving: 127.6

Carbs: 13g

Protein: 7.2g

Fat: 5.2g

Glazed Ribs

Preparation time: 10 minutes

Cooking time: 1 hour and 20 minutes

Servings: 4

Ingredients:

1 rack pork ribs, ribs separated

1 and ¼ cups tomato sauce

¼ cup white vinegar

3 tablespoons spicy mustard

2 tablespoons coconut sugar

3 tablespoons water

¼ teaspoon hot sauce

1 teaspoon onion powder

Cooking spray

Directions:

Put the ribs in a baking dish, cover with tin foil and bake in the oven at 400 degrees F for 1 hour.

Heat up a pan with the tomato sauce, mustard, sugar, vinegar, water, onion powder and hot sauce, stir, cook for 10 minutes and take off heat. Baste the ribs with half of this sauce, place them on preheated grill over medium-high heat, grease them with cooking spray, cook for 4 minutes on each side, divide between plates and serve with the rest of the sauce on the side.

Enjoy!

Nutrition:

Calories 287,

Fat 5,

Fiber 8,

Carbs 16,

Protein 15

Sodium 72%

Tavern Sandwiches in Instant Pot

Preparation time: 5 minutes

Cook Time: 15 minutes

Serves: 8

Ingredients:

2 pounds ground beef

½ teaspoon salt

10 oz. Can chicken gumbo soup with a little bit of liquid left

2 tablespoons mustard

8 slices American cheese

3 chopped green onions

¼ teaspoon pepper

1 can tomato soup

1 tablespoon ketchup

Split sandwich buns

Directions:

Press sauté button on instant pot and cook ground beef till it's not pink.

Add all ingredients but the cheese and bun, cooking it on high for 7 minutes.

Quick release it, and spoon it into a bun, adding cheese to serve.

Nutrition:

Calories: 270,

Fat: 10g

Carbs: 22gNet

Carbs: 17g

Protein: 20g

Fiber: 5g

Sodium 67%

Tuscan Chicken Pasta

Preparation time: 10 minutes

Cook Time: 4 minutes

Servings: 6

Ingredients:

  3 cups low-Sodium chicken broth

  ½ tablespoon Italian seasoning

  12 oz. Whole wheat noodles

  1 cup cottage cheese

  ¼ teaspoon pepper

  1/3 cup sun-dried tomatoes

  1 tablespoon minced garlic

  2 pounds chicken breast

  2 cups spinach

  1 cup plain Greek yogurt

  ¼ cup Parmesan

  ¼ cup basil

Directions:

Turn IP onto sauté and add the tomatoes, garlic, seasoning pepper, and salt, stirring for 30 seconds.

Add the chicken and brown for 1-2 minutes and keep the chicken from sticking. add pasta and chicken broth and stir to cover it.

Manual cook it for 4 minutes, and then quick release the pressure, but be careful. Blend the yogurt and cottage cheese and set it aside.

Stir pasta and noodles, and then add cheese, basil, and spinach, and mix it till everything is combined.

Pour cream over pasta, and then stir till all is covered.

Nutrition:

Calories: 479

Fat: 9g Carbs: 49gNet Carbs: 48g Protein: 54g Fiber: 1g Sodium 52%

Chinese Chicken

Preparation time: 10 minutes,

Cook Time: 10 minutes

Serves: 4

Ingredients:

5 pounds chicken thighs

½ cup balsamic vinegar

1 teaspoon dried black peppercorns

½ cup coconut amino

black pepper for taste

4 cloves minced garlic.

Directions:

Within the instant pot, mix chicken with vinegar, amino, garlic, pepper, and the peppercorns. Mix it together.

Then, cook it on high for 15 minutes.

Divide it, and then serve!

Nutrition:

Calories 261,

Fat 7g

Carbs 18gNet

Carbs: 10g

Protein: 8g

Fiber 8g

Sodium 33%

Bell Peppers 'n Tomato-Chickpea Rice

Preparation Time: 35 minutes

Cooking Time: 35 minutes

Servings: 4

Ingredients:

2 tablespoons olive oil

1/2 chopped red bell pepper

1/2 chopped green bell pepper

1/2 chopped yellow pepper

1/2 chopped red pepper

1 medium onion, chopped

1 clove garlic, minced

2 cups cooked jasmine rice

1 teaspoon tomato paste

1 cup chickpeas

salt to taste

1/2 teaspoon paprika

1 small tomato, chopped

Parsley for garnish

Directions:

In a large mixing bowl, whisk well olive oil, garlic, tomato paste, and paprika. Season with salt generously. Mix in rice and toss well to coat in the dressing. Add remaining ingredients and toss well to mix.

Let salad rest to allow flavors to mix for 15 minutes.

Toss one more time and adjust salt to taste if needed.

Garnish with parsley and serve.

Nutrition:

Calories per serving: 490

Carbs: 93.0g

Protein: 10.0g

Fat: 8.0g

Avocado and Turkey Mix Panini

Preparation Time: 8 minutes

Cooking Time: 8 minutes

Servings: 2

Ingredients:

- 2 red peppers, roasted and sliced into strips
- ¼ lb. thinly sliced mesquite smoked turkey breast
- 1 cup whole fresh spinach leaves, divided
- 2 slices provolone cheese
- 1 tbsp olive oil, divided
- 2 ciabatta rolls
- ¼ cup mayonnaise
- ½ ripe avocado

Directions:

In a bowl, mash thoroughly together mayonnaise and avocado. Then preheat Panini press.

Slice the bread rolls in half and spread olive oil on the insides of the bread. Then fill it with filling, layering them as you go: provolone, turkey breast, roasted red pepper, spinach leaves and spread avocado mixture and cover with the other bread slice.

Place sandwich in the Panini press and grill for 5 to 8 minutes until cheese has melted and bread is crisped and ridged.

Nutrition:

- Calories per Serving: 546
- Carbs: 31.9g
- Protein: 27.8g
- Fat: 34.8g

Black Bean Enchilada Skillet Casserole

Preparation Time: 15 minutes

Cooking Time: 15 minutes

Servings: 6

Ingredients:

1 tablespoon extra-virgin olive oil

½ onion, chopped

½ red bell pepper, seeded and chopped

½ green bell pepper, seeded and chopped

2 small zucchinis, chopped

3 garlic cloves, minced

1 (15-ounce) can low-sodium black beans, drained and rinsed

1 (10-ounce) can low-sodium enchilada sauce

1 teaspoon ground cumin

¼ teaspoon salt

¼ teaspoon freshly ground black pepper

½ cup shredded cheddar cheese, divided

2 (6-inch) corn tortillas, cut into strips

Chopped fresh cilantro, for garnish

Plain yogurt, for serving

Directions:

Heat the broiler to high.

In a large oven-safe skillet, heat the oil over medium-high heat.

Add the onion, red bell pepper, green bell pepper, zucchini, and garlic to the skillet, and cook for 3 to 5 minutes until the onion softens.

Add the black beans, enchilada sauce, cumin, salt, pepper, ¼ cup of cheese, and tortilla strips, and mix together. Top with the remaining ¼ cup of cheese.

Put the skillet under the broiler and broil for 5 to 8 minutes until the cheese is melted and bubbly. Garnish with cilantro and serve with yogurt on the side.

Nutrition:
Calories: 171
Total Fat: 7g
Protein: 8g
Carbohydrates: 21g
Sugars: 3g
Fiber: 7g
Sodium: 565mg

Crispy Parmesan Cups with White Beans and Veggies

Preparation Time: 10 minutes

Cooking Time: 5 minutes

Servings: 4

Ingredients:

1 cup grated Parmesan cheese, divided

1 (15-ounce) can low-sodium white beans, drained and rinsed

1 cucumber, peeled and finely diced

½ cup finely diced red onion

¼ cup thinly sliced fresh basil

1 garlic clove, minced

½ jalapeño pepper, diced

1 tablespoon extra-virgin olive oil

1 tablespoon balsamic vinegar

¼ teaspoon salt

Freshly ground black pepper

Directions:

Heat a medium nonstick skillet over medium heat. Sprinkle 2 tablespoons of cheese in a thin circle in the center of the pan, flattening it with a spatula. When the cheese melts, use a spatula to flip the cheese and lightly brown the other side. Remove the cheese "pancake" from the pan and place into the cup of a muffin tin, bending it gently with your hands to fit in the muffin cup.

Repeat with the remaining cheese until you have 8 cups.

In a mixing bowl, combine the beans, cucumber, onion, basil, garlic, jalapeño, olive oil, and vinegar, and season with the salt and pepper.

Nutrition:

Calories: 259; Total Fat: 12g; Protein: 15g; Carbohydrates: 24g; Sugars: 4g; Fiber: 8g; Sodium: 551mg

Brussels Sprout, Avocado, and Wild Rice Bowl

Preparation Time: 15 minutes

Cooking Time: 15 minutes

Servings: 4

Ingredients:

  2 cups sliced Brussels sprouts

  2 teaspoons extra-virgin olive oil, plus 2 tablespoons

  Juice of 1 lemon

  1 teaspoon Dijon mustard

  1 garlic clove, minced

  ½ teaspoon salt

  ¼ teaspoon freshly ground black pepper

  1 cup cooked wild rice

  1 cup sliced radishes

  1 avocado, sliced

Directions:

Preheat the oven to 400°F. Line a baking sheet with parchment paper.

In a medium bowl, toss the Brussels sprouts with 2 teaspoons of olive oil and spread on the prepared baking sheet. Roast for 12 minutes, stirring once, until lightly browned.

In a small bowl, mix the remaining 2 tablespoons of olive oil, lemon juice, mustard, garlic, salt, and pepper.

In a large bowl, toss the cooked wild rice, radishes, and roasted Brussels sprouts. Drizzle the dressing over the salad and toss.

Divide among 4 bowls and top with avocado slices.

Nutrition:

  Calories: 178; Total Fat: 11g; Protein: 2g; Carbohydrates: 18g; Sugars: 2g; Fiber: 5g; Sodium: 299mg

Sweet Potato, Chickpea, and Kale Bowl with Creamy Tahini Sauce

Preparation Time: 10 minutes

Cooking Time: 15 minutes

Servings: 2

Ingredients:

2 tablespoons plain nonfat Greek yogurt

1 tablespoon tahini

2 tablespoons hemp seeds

1 garlic clove, minced

Pinch salt

Freshly ground black pepper

FOR THE BOWL

1 small sweet potato, peeled and finely diced

1 teaspoon extra-virgin olive oil

1 cup from 1 (15-ounce) can low-sodium chickpeas, drained and rinsed

2 cups baby kale

Directions:

TO MAKE THE SAUCE

In a small bowl, whisk together the yogurt and tahini.

Stir in the hemp seeds, garlic, and salt. Season with pepper. Add 2 to 3 tablespoons water to create a creamy yet pourable consistency. Set aside.

TO MAKE THE BOWL

Preheat the oven to 425°F. Line a baking sheet with parchment paper.

Arrange the sweet potato on the prepared baking sheet and drizzle with the olive oil. Toss. Roast for 10 to 15 minutes, stirring once, until tender and browned.

In each of 2 bowls, arrange ½ cup of chickpeas, 1 cup of kale, and half of the cooked sweet potato. Drizzle with half the creamy tahini sauce and serve.

Nutrition:

Calories: 322; Total Fat: 14g; Protein: 17g; Carbohydrates: 36g; Sugars: 7g; Fiber: 8g; Sodium: 305mg

Baked Tofu and Mixed Vegetable Bowl

Preparation Time: 10 minutes

Cooking Time: 20 minutes

Servings: 4

Ingredients:

Nonstick cooking spray

1 (14-ounce) container firm tofu, cut into 1½-inch cubes

2 tablespoons low-sodium gluten-free soy sauce or tamari

1 tablespoon toasted sesame oil

1 teaspoon grated fresh ginger

1 teaspoon honey

2 garlic cloves, minced

2 teaspoons cornstarch

¼ cup water, plus 2 tablespoons

2 teaspoons extra-virgin olive oil

2 cups thinly sliced bokchoy

1 cup sliced shiitake mushrooms

1 cup thinly sliced carrots

1 (14-ounce) can baby corn, drained and rinsed

4 scallions, both white and green parts, chopped

Directions:

Preheat the oven to 400°F. Line a baking sheet with parchment paper. Spray the parchment paper with nonstick cooking spray.

Place the tofu cubes on the prepared baking sheet and bake for 20 minutes, flipping once, until they are browned.

In a small bowl, combine the soy sauce, sesame oil, ginger, honey, and garlic. Stir well to combine.

In another small bowl, mix the cornstarch with ¼ cup of water and stir to combine. Add the soy sauce mixture, stir together, and set aside.

In a large skillet, heat the oil over medium heat. Add the boy choy, mushrooms, and carrots, and cook for 3 minutes, stirring regularly.

Add the remaining 2 tablespoons of water, cover, and steam the vegetables for 3 more minutes until just fork-tender. Add the baby corn.

Pour the sauce and cooked tofu into the skillet and bring to a boil. Reduce the heat and simmer for 1 to 2 minutes until the sauce thickens.

Divide the tofu and vegetables among 4 bowls. Top with scallions and serve.

Nutrition:

Calories: 212; Total Fat: 11g; Protein: 12g; Carbohydrates: 22g; Sugars: 7g; Fiber: 4g; Sodium: 526mg

Mozzarella and Artichoke Stuffed Spaghetti Squash

Preparation Time: 10 minutes

Cooking Time: 45 minutes

Servings: 4

Ingredients:

1 small spaghetti squash, halved and seeded

½ cup low-fat cottage cheese

¼ cup shredded mozzarella cheese, divided

2 garlic cloves, minced

1 cup artichoke hearts, chopped

1 cup thinly sliced kale

⅛ teaspoon salt

Pinch freshly ground black pepper

Directions:

Preheat the oven to 400°F. Line a baking sheet with parchment paper. Place the cut squash halves on the prepared baking sheet cut-side down, and roast for 30 to 40 minutes, depending on the size and thickness of the squash, until they are fork-tender. Set aside to cool slightly. In a large bowl, mix the cottage cheese, 2 tablespoons of mozzarella cheese, garlic, artichoke hearts, kale, salt, and pepper.

Preheat the broiler to high. Using a fork, break apart the flesh of the spaghetti squash into strands, being careful to leave the skin intact. Add the strands to the cheese and vegetable mixture. Toss gently to combine. Divide the mixture between the two hollowed-out squash halves and top with the remaining 2 tablespoons of cheese. Broil for 5 to 7 minutes until browned and heated through.

Cut each piece of stuffed squash in half to serve.

Nutrition:

Calories: 142; Total Fat: 4g; Protein: 9g; Carbohydrates: 19g; Sugars: 10g; Fiber: 4g; Sodium: 312mg

Mushroom Cutlets with Creamy Sauce

Preparation Time: 15 minutes

Cooking Time: 20 minutes

Servings: 4

Ingredients:

FOR THE SAUCE

1 tablespoon extra-virgin olive oil

2 tablespoons whole-wheat flour

1½ cups unsweetened plain almond milk

¼ teaspoon salt

Dash Worcestershire sauce

Pinch cayenne pepper

¼ cup shredded cheddar cheese

FOR THE CUTLETS

2 eggs

2 cups chopped mushrooms

1 cup quick oats

2 scallions, both white and green parts, chopped

¼ cup shredded cheddar cheese

½ teaspoon salt

¼ teaspoon freshly ground black pepper

1 tablespoon extra-virgin olive oil

Directions:

TO MAKE THE SAUCE

1.In a medium saucepan, heat the oil over medium heat. Add the flour and stir constantly for about 2 minutes until browned.

2.Slowly whisk in the almond milk and bring to a boil. Reduce the heat to low and simmer for 6 to 8 minutes until the sauce thickens.

3.Season with the salt, Worcestershire sauce, and cayenne. Add the cheese and stir until melted. Turn off the heat and cover to keep warm while you make the cutlets.

TO MAKE THE CUTLETS

1.In a large mixing bowl, beat the eggs. Add the mushrooms, oats, scallions, cheese, salt, and pepper. Stir to combine.

2.Using your hands, form the mixture into 8 patties, each about ½ inch thick.

3.In a large skillet, heat the oil over medium-high heat. Cook the patties, in batches if necessary, for 3 minutes per side until crisp and brown.

4.Serve the cutlets warm with sauce drizzled over the top.

Nutrition:

Calories: 261; Total Fat: 17g; Protein: 11g; Carbohydrates: 18g; Sugars: 2g; Fiber: 3g; Sodium: 559mg

Falafel with Creamy Garlic-Yogurt Sauce

Preparation Time: 15 minutes

Cooking Time: 10 minutes

Servings: 4

Ingredients:

FOR THE SAUCE

¾ cup plain nonfat Greek yogurt

3 garlic cloves, minced

Juice of 1 lemon

1 tablespoon extra-virgin olive oil

¼ teaspoon salt

FOR THE FALAFEL

1 (15-ounce) can low-sodium chickpeas, drained and rinsed

2 garlic cloves, roughly chopped

2 tablespoons whole-wheat flour

2 tablespoons chopped fresh parsley

½ teaspoon ground cumin

¼ teaspoon salt

2 teaspoons canola oil, divided

8 large lettuce leaves, chopped

1 cucumber, chopped

1 tomato, diced

Directions:

TO MAKE THE SAUCE

In a small bowl, combine the yogurt, garlic, lemon juice, olive oil, and salt, and mix well. Cover and refrigerate until ready to serve.

TO MAKE THE FALAFEL

In a food processor or blender, combine the chickpeas and garlic, and pulse until chopped well but not creamy. Add the flour, parsley, cumin, and salt. Pulse several more times until incorporated.

Using your hands, form the mixture into balls, using about 1 tablespoon of mixture for each ball.

In a medium skillet, heat 1 teaspoon of canola oil over medium-high heat. Working in batches, add the falafel to the skillet, cooking on each side for 2 to 3 minutes until browned and crisp. Remove the falafel from the skillet and repeat with the remaining oil and falafel until all are cooked.

Divide the lettuce, cucumber, and tomato among 4 plates.

Top each plate with 2 falafel and 2 tablespoons of sauce. Serve immediately.

Nutrition:

Calories: 219; Total Fat: 8g; Protein: 12g; Carbohydrates: 27g; Sugars: 6g; Fiber: 7g; Sodium: 462mg

Thai-Style Chicken Soup

Preparation Time: 10 minutes

Cooking Time: 15 minutes

Servings: 4

Ingredients:

1 tablespoon vegetable oil

1 small onion, thinly sliced

2 garlic cloves, minced

2 tablespoons red curry paste

4 cups low-sodium chicken broth

1 (15-ounce) can lite coconut milk

1½ cups sugar snap or snow peas, sliced lengthwise

4 ounces vermicelli rice noodles, broken into pieces

1-pound boneless skinless chicken breast, thinly sliced

1 tablespoon fish sauce

2 teaspoons brown sugar

Juice of 1 lime

1 lime, cut into wedges

Handful fresh basil leaves, chopped

Directions:

In a large pot over medium-high heat, heat the vegetable oil.

Add the onion, and cook for 5 to 7 minutes, until softened and starting to brown.

Add the garlic and curry paste, and cook, stirring, for about 1 minute, until fragrant.

Stir in the chicken broth and coconut milk and bring to a boil. Reduce the heat to maintain a simmer and add the peas and noodles. Cook for about 3 minutes, until the noodles are just barely tender.

Add the chicken and simmer for 3 minutes, until cooked through.

Season with the fish sauce, brown sugar, and lime juice. Divide among bowls and serve with lime wedges and topped with basil.

Nutrition:

Calories: 372; Total fat: 13g; Saturated fat: 6g; Protein: 33g; Carbs: 32g; Sugar: 3g; Fiber: 2g; Cholesterol: 65mg; Sodium: 912mg

Herb-Roasted Chicken Breast

Preparation Time: 5 minutes

Cooking Time: 25 minutes

Servings: 4-6

Ingredients:

1 tablespoon extra-virgin olive oil

1 teaspoon chopped fresh thyme

½ teaspoon dried oregano

½ teaspoon garlic powder

½ teaspoon onion powder

½ teaspoon salt

4 boneless skinless chicken breasts

Directions:

Preheat the oven to 400°F.

In a small bowl, stir together the olive oil, thyme, oregano, garlic powder, onion powder, and salt.

Place the chicken breasts on a baking sheet or in a baking dish, and rub both sides with the herb mixture. Leave a couple of inches between each breast. Bake for 20 to 25 minutes, until the juices run clear and the internal temperature measures 165°F on an instant-read thermometer.

Let the chicken rest for 5 minutes before slicing and serving.

Nutrition:

Calories: 153; Total fat: 5g; Saturated fat: 1g; Protein: 26g; Carbs: 1g; Sugar: 0g; Fiber: 0g; Cholesterol: 65mg; Sodium: 366mg

HOW EASY IS MEDITERRANEAN DIET TO FOLLOW?

To begin on the Mediterranean diet plan, the principal thing you should do is dispensing with the red meat from your day by day menu. While you can have it every so often, it shouldn't be something you eat habitually by any stretch of the imagination. From that point, start centring the base of your diet around entire grains, organic products, vegetables, nuts, and seeds. Add fish and seafood to one meal daily, just as chicken, eggs, cheddar, and yoghurt once per day or each other day. Sheep is additionally usually found in this diet. However, it is treated as an irregularity. Changing the diet mentality can be more testing than one may suspect. Following a specific program for weight, misfortune might be sufficiently sound if the plan is wealthy in nutritious foods that are adjusted and fulfilling.

Notwithstanding, regardless of whether it is the most nutritionally stable program on the planet if that program doesn't show you how to change propensities, practices, and decisions for your lifetime, it will just add up to simply one more diet that has travelled every which way, weight loss, weight picked up once more. How would we figure out how to roll out the improvements essential for a lifetime and not one minute in time, and for what reason do these progressions appear to be so troublesome and slippery?

We should look at four of the best and significant changes you can make that will endure forever and keep the additional weight off for good, since dear peruser, the characteristic of a really effective "diet" is the one that shows you how never to recover it again. Regardless of whether you've shed pounds previously and restored it again, or just picked up and never lost, whichever way reality of progress lies in the life change.

Ensure that you are eating routinely to keep your blood glucose levels balanced out and hunger level under wraps. Three principle meals, in addition to a few snacks for each day, will work best for most by far from individuals. Wean yourself off any desserts you might be eating. Note that you may get yourself a few desserts that you appreciate now and again just, yet separated from that, they ought to be avoided. The Mediterranean diet is a nutritional model inspired by the habits of the European countries of the Mediterranean Sea basin.

The main ingredients of this diet are olive oil, wine, fish, cereals, white meats, dairy products, eggs, fruits and vegetables. The Mediterranean diet consists of a healthy and balanced diet. From a nutritional point of view, it is able to reduce the incidence of diseases of different kinds, namely: diabetes, cardiovascular diseases and tumours, as well as recent studies show that it would be able to slow down the cognitive decline caused by ageing.

You should know that the word "Mediterranean diet" goes beyond simple nutrition; it identifies a real lifestyle, which includes gastronomic, agricultural, popular traditions and various relationships between different cultures. The Mediterranean diet is a sustainable diet not only for human health but also for the environment itself. In fact, thanks to the use of mainly natural resources, it combats greenhouse gas emissions, guaranteeing the consumption of products while respecting their seasonality and biodiversity.

Don't follow the old rule that you should only shop the perimeter of the grocery store. Today's supermarkets have Mediterranean Diet staples in every aisle—including the middle ones. While shopping, picture the Mediterranean Diet Pyramid inside your shopping cart: Half your cart should be fruits, vegetables, and plant-based foods, then fill up the rest with seafood, and so on.

The Mediterranean diet is meant to be followed long term; therefore, the meal plan given in this part is designed to help you kickstart your journey. The meal plan was created with the 100 recipes listed in the books. The recipes are flexible and can be rotated among the days as you please. This is the beginning of your journey, note that you will need a lot of discipline and dedication to continue after the 31 days planned for you. That is when the spirit of diversity and experimentation has to come in. You have to be able to search for dishes online and combine a couple of them to make your very own recipes.

THE MEDITERRANEAN DIET PYRAMID

As illustrated in the pyramid, fresh fruits and vegetables, grains such as whole-wheat bread, pasta, or rice, and olive oil are important parts of every meal. Foods enjoyed daily include nuts, cheese, or yogurt, and red wine. Fish, eggs, poultry, and legumes are consumed several times a week, and meat is restricted to a few times a month.

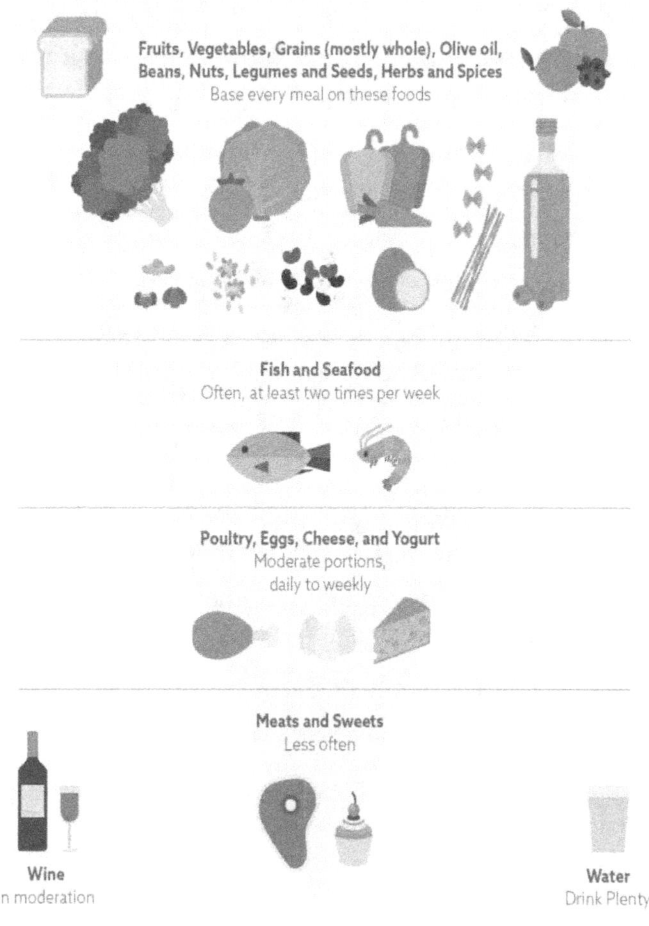

Kick-Start Your Mediterranean Diet

The Mediterranean diet has been carried out with great success by people around the world. This diet contributes to weight loss, maintains healthy weight and improves overall health by switching bad fats to nutrient-dense foods and making small lifestyle changes.

Together we'll explore the basics of the Mediterranean diet, including how it relates to nutrition, exercise, and portion control, and how you can easily apply it to your lifestyle. You'll learn how to shop and cook like a true yiayia. And although this book contains many

Mediterranean specialties, you'll quickly see that this cooking style isn't so foreign. At its roots, the Mediterranean diet is about whole foods that come from the earth and are available in most grocery stores. It's not exotic cooking—it's good, healthy cooking!

Friends and family—from novices to experienced cooks—helped us test the recipes in this book. While each of these recipes takes around 30 minutes or less, keep in mind that the prep and cooking times are our best estimates. Different people (and different ovens) do things at different speeds. And we often are prepping ingredients while something is cooking in the oven or on the stove, which is reflected in the cooking times.

We always recommend that you first read the recipe all the way through and get all your ingredients out before diving in. This will ultimately save you time in the kitchen—and make sure your dinner is done in around 30 minutes or less!

If you're cooking for family or guests with varied tastes or special dietary needs, we've got you covered. Look for the following labels:

Dairy-free

Nut-free

Gluten-free

Egg-free

Vegetarian

Vegan

5 ingredients (not including water, salt, pepper, oil, and nonstick cooking spray)

One pot (the recipe can be cooked in a single pot or pan or baking dish)

Half the time (15 minutes or less from start to finish, including all the prep and cooking)

Remember to always check labels while you shop, though. For example, some ingredients like oats are naturally gluten-free but processed in factories with cross contamination. If gluten or nuts are a concern for you, be sure to look out for labels on packaging before you buy or use anything.

And if you remember only one thing, remember this: The Mediterranean Diet is NOT a strict diet.

It's a pattern of eating based on vegetables, fruits, whole grains, fish, beans, nuts, olive oil, and some dairy and meat. Please swap ingredients in and out of our recipes based on your preferences.

What we mean is, use brown rice if you don't have quinoa. Use spinach if you don't like kale. Almonds will work instead of walnuts. And even though some produce (pineapples), whole grains (wild rice), nuts (pecans), and seafood (salmon) aren't really grown or harvested in the Mediterranean region, that doesn't mean you shouldn't happily swap them into recipes to make them your own.

One last note: Make this book messy! Dog-ear the pages and write notes in the margins. These recipes are a starting place to build your confidence in cooking the Mediterranean way, using what you have on hand and what tastes good to you and your family.

KNOW YOUR BODY FOR INTUITIVE EATING

It's easy to be healthy when you live in a sunny country on the Mediterranean Sea. With the ocean breeze, sunshine, and good wine, how could you be stressed out and lack energy? Part of the Mediterranean Diet means adopting a bit of a vacation-mode attitude, at least for several minutes throughout the day. Here's how:

Slow down at mealtimes. Time the length of one of your regular family meals. Then, try stretching it out just 10 minutes longer, to include conversation with the folks at your table. And yes, please eat at a table with all TVs, phones, and electronics off. You'll be on your way to the relaxed meal that's a signature of Mediterranean regions.

Savor a glass of wine. Savoring wine with a meal helps slow down your dinners. Serve wine (it doesn't have to be an expensive bottle) on the nights you have time to appreciate it or serve it with a leisurely lunch on the weekends. It's customary to enjoy wine only when food is also being served.

The Mediterranean diet concentrates on traditional foods and recipes that can be found in Mediterranean-style cooking. This is what's going on in the Mediterranean diet. This includes eating lots of vegetables and grains, fruit, rice and pasta while reducing fats, substituting salt with spices and herbs, and eat fish and chicken instead of processed meats. There is not a lot of red meat in the Mediterranean diet. Nuts are part of a healthy part of the diet. One should, however, limit oneself to a handful or so a day. Nuts have a high-fat content, but a high-fat content is not saturated.

Nuts are also high in calories, so carefully monitor the amount you eat. You'll want to avoid salted nuts and honey roasted or candied nuts.

It may even include a glass of red wine per day and regular physical activity to fully maximize remarkable health benefits. The Western diet illustrates the diverse eating habits of countries near to the

Mediterranean coast, mainly southern Italy, Greece, Morocco, France and Spain. Due to its unique location, the climate encourages fresh fruit, vegetables and some of the best seafood in the world.

This diet isn't focused on limiting your total consumption of fat. Instead, it focuses on making smarter choices about the kinds of fat you consume. This diet discourages people from eating trans-fats and saturated fats, both of which have been linked to heart disease.

Move that body more often. You could have the healthiest diet in the world, but without moving your muscles, your body won't be truly fit. Keeping your muscles strong helps prevent injured backs and shoulders and makes it easier to do just about everything. Think of daily physical activity as insurance against aches and pains. It is also an amazing way to relieve stress. Even 10-minute spurts of activity several times throughout the day lead to better health.

Get a good night's sleep. Aim for seven to eight hours of sleep nightly. We can't stress this enough. We know people who have changed their entire lives just by regularly getting enough sleep. Even with the best diet and exercise plan in the world, your body will not work as efficiently without enough sleep. Make it a priority.

CONCLUSION

It's important to note that the Mediterranean diet isn't just about diet - it's a lifestyle change. You will be focusing on eating a diet with less red meat and more fresh fruits, vegetables, and seafood, but if you truly want to mimic the lifestyle of the Mediterranean, you have to incorporate physical activity into your routine. The people of this region naturally fit exercise into their daily lives whether it was through walking, swimming, or boating. To gain the same health benefits, you should try and be more active in your life to gain those similar health benefits. Even if you aren't going to the gym, try and make more conscious choices to burn calories and get your body moving. You could take a walk around the block, jog, or bike, or spend some time gardening. Simply making the decision to be more active allows you to expend calories and lose more weight.

We provided a detailed look at the Mediterranean lifestyle and exactly what it entails. The more informed you are about this diet and exactly what you should and should not be eating, the greater your chances of success will be! We've shared about the history behind the Mediterranean diet and how the research proves the many multiple health benefits this diet can provide. People who go Mediterranean can lose more weight, lower their risk factors of heart disease, and even preserve your bone mass and muscle mass later in life! By keeping your cells more active and healthier, you can slow down the process of aging that affects all of us over time. There can be a few disadvantages to the Mediterranean diet that people have to adjust to, but with the many health benefits, it's obvious that the good outweighs the bad. Without the need to count calories or weigh your portion sizes, the ease of flexibility this diet provides makes it so appealing to many.

To help you succeed, we have included many tips for weight loss and how to implement the Mediterranean diet into your lifestyle long-term. It's important you know exactly what habits and foods you should be incorporating in your routine, like staying hydrated, having a diet full of fiber, and planning a mealtime schedule to avoid excess snacking. The more you are able to sustain a healthy diet, the less likely you will be to reach for the "forbidden" items like sugary snacks, processed foods, soda, or candy. It is important you remind yourself of all the things you can eat on the Mediterranean diet versus what you cannot eat. There are so many varieties of food you can include in your meals like vegetables, whole grains, fish, seafood, beans, and even fruit! Some diets restrict fruit due to their natural sugars and net carbs, but the Mediterranean diet urges you to use fruit to satisfy your sweet tooth! You can even have your glass of your favorite wine if you are a wine drinker, but it's important you speak to your physician to ensure that you can drink alcohol with your individual health needs and condition. We hope you enjoy this cookbook!

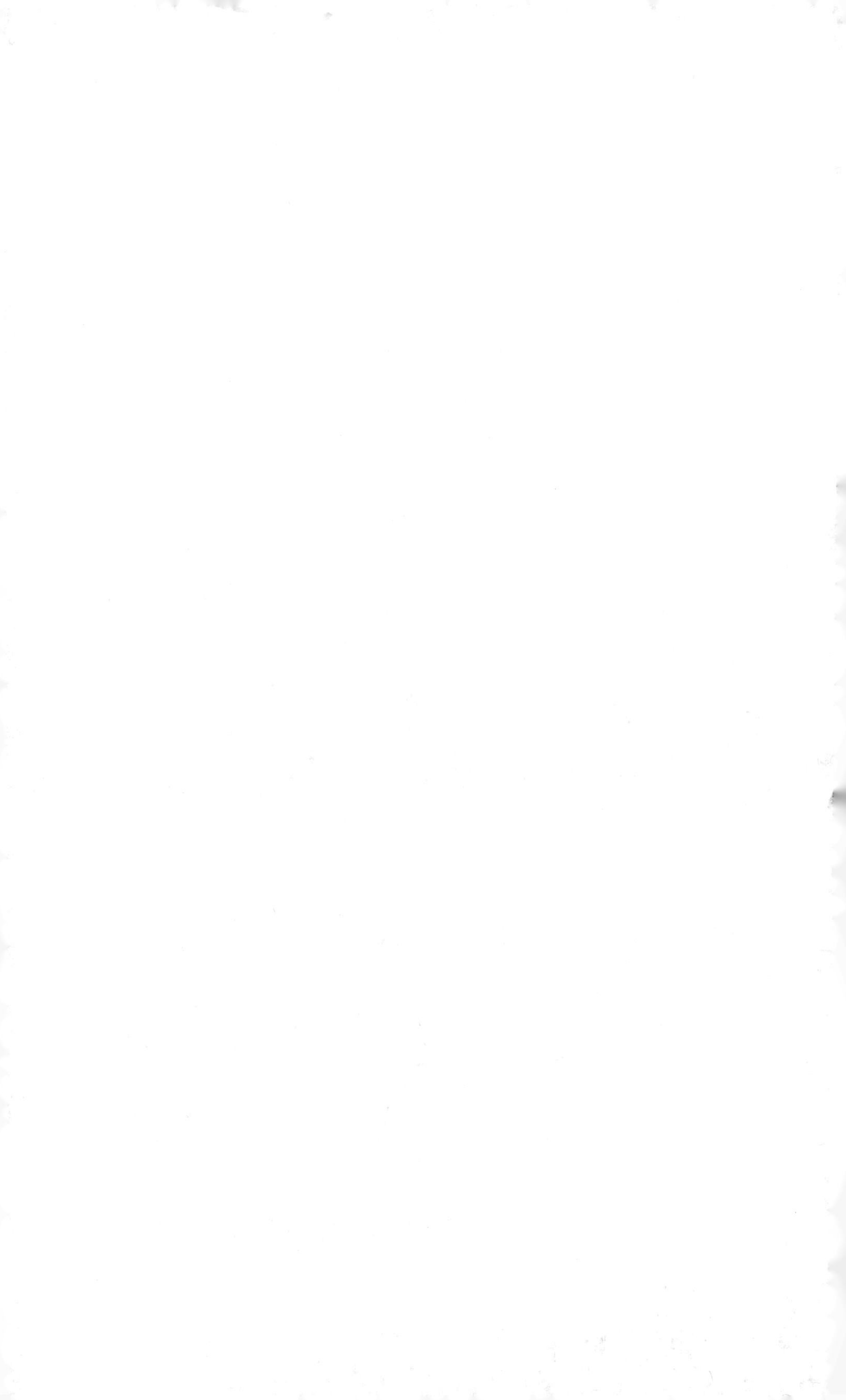